AF680554

# THE FIRST-YEAR NURSE'S SURVIVAL GUIDE

## *Lessons & Stories for New Graduates and Foreign-Trained Nurses*

BY

PIA DY,
MSN, RN, PCCN

Copyright © 2025 by Pia Dy. All right reserved.

No part of this publication may be reproduced, distributed, or transmitted in any form or by any means, including photocopying, recording, or other electronic or mechanical methods, without prior written permission of the author, except in the case of brief quotations in critical reviews and certain other noncommercial uses permitted by copyright law.

Published by Pia Dy
Westchester County, New York, USA

eBook Edition

ISBN: (Assigned by KDP)

Cover design by Pia Dy

Interior design by Pia Dy

This book is a work of creative nonfiction. Some names and identifying details have been changed to protect privacy.

# Contents

# PREFACE

## The Choice and the Crossing

There are moments that divide a life, the instant before a decision, and the long path that follows.

For me, that moment began quietly, in the small hours of a humid Manila night, when the house was still and my mind refused to rest. I sat on the edge of my bed, staring at an open suitcase that already felt too small to hold everything I loved. My stethoscope lay beside folded scrubs, the metal cool against my fingers a reminder of what I was leaving and what I was reaching for.

I had spent years caring for other people's families while my own dreams waited in the corners of my heart. Now a choice stood in front of me: stay close to my son and continue a life that was safe but limited, or step into the unknown thousands of miles away in search of something better. It wasn't ambition that kept me awake that night; it was fear. Fear that leaving would break something sacred, and fear that staying would break something in me.

The world outside was dark, yet I could hear the faint hum of the city: distant traffic, a dog barking, a neighbor's radio playing an old love song. Each sound felt like a goodbye. I watched the first light of morning spread across the wall and thought of my son still asleep, his small hand curled against his cheek. How do you tell a child that love sometimes means leaving?

That question has followed me for years. It was the beginning of a journey that would test my faith, my endurance, and the very definition of home.

When people ask why I became a nurse, I tell them it began long before I held a license. It began with a hunger to serve, to heal, to make meaning out of struggle. But the truth is, nursing found me through loss. It asked for everything time, strength, and pieces of my heart I didn't know I could give.

The day I finally boarded that plane, I thought the hardest part was over. I believed the struggle would be external adapting to a new country, a new system, a new life. I didn't yet understand that the real challenge would be internal: learning how to belong in a world that didn't yet have a place for me.

That realization didn't come in a grand moment. It crept in quietly, through the exhaustion of night shifts and the weight of unfamiliar expectations. There were days I moved through hallways filled with noise and still felt invisible. There were nights when silence was heavier than any workload. Yet, in those same moments, I also discovered a kind of faith that no church had ever taught me the faith that purpose is often hidden inside pain.

It was during one of those long nights that I began to see my life differently. I was no longer a woman who had left home; I was a woman building a new one. Every patient I cared for, every colleague who offered a kind word, every lesson that humbled me they all became part of that home.

## The Realization and the Promise

Years passed before I understood that healing others was also healing me. Each small victory the smile of a patient who finally slept, the hand squeezed in gratitude, the quiet moment when fear turned to trust stitched a new layer of meaning into the choice I once feared would break me.

There were setbacks too: days when nothing went right, when I questioned whether all the sacrifice had been worth it. Yet even in those moments, purpose whispered through the noise. It reminded me that nursing is not a single act of care but a lifelong practice of becoming.

As my career grew and I stepped into the role of an educator, I began to see the same uncertainty I once carried reflected in the faces of new nurses. They arrived with the same mix of fear and hope eager to help but afraid to fail. Watching them was like looking into a mirror that showed my past and my promise at once.

That realization changed how I taught. I stopped focusing only on what they needed to know and started teaching them what they needed to believe: that compassion has power, that mistakes can be teachers, and that strength often begins as self-doubt. I wanted them to understand that the real lessons of nursing live not in textbooks, but in the quiet spaces between exhaustion and grace.

Writing this book was an extension of that teaching. I wanted to gather the lessons that had shaped me the sleepless nights, the laughter shared in break rooms, the stories that lingered long after the shift ended and place them in the hands of those just beginning their own journey. I wanted this book to be a light carried forward, one nurse at a time.

When I look back now, I realize that the greatest struggle was never leaving home; it was learning to create belonging wherever I stood. The hospital corridors, once foreign, became familiar. The colleagues who started as strangers became family. And the woman who once doubted she could endure became someone who helps others find their strength.

This is what nursing has taught me: that courage is not the absence of fear, but the decision to keep showing up. It is found in the small moments the steadying breath before a difficult task, the calm voice in chaos, the kindness offered when you have little left to give.

I have written these pages for every nurse standing at the threshold of their first year, for every foreign-trained nurse building a life far from home, and for every caregiver who wonders if their effort is enough. You are not alone.

If this book finds you in a moment of uncertainty, let it remind you that your struggle is proof of your growth. Every challenge you face is preparing you for the nurse and the person you are becoming.

And so, before you turn the page, know this: you are already part of a legacy. The courage that brought you here will carry you forward. The same strength that once guided me now belongs to you.

*This is my promise to you that within these pages, you will find echoes of your own story, reminders of your worth, and the assurance that even on the hardest days, you are never walking alone.*

Before we begin, let me take you back to the moment my own story truly started to unfold.

# INTRODUCTION

Every nurse has a beginning.

Mine started with two suitcases, a passport, and twenty dollars in my pocket. I left the Philippines not as a tourist but as a mother chasing a promise one, I had whispered to my seven-year-old son, Liam: that one day he would join me in America, and I would build a life sturdy enough to hold both of our dreams.

What I didn't know then was that every dream worth chasing comes with a cost. Mine was measured in distance and silence in birthdays I would miss, in good-night calls cut short by time zones, in the quiet ache of a mother learning to love from miles away.

The flight to Newark stretched nineteen hours and felt endless. Every minute carried a different weight: hope, fear, guilt, faith. I replayed each goodbye Liam's small hands clinging to mine at the airport, my sister's steady eyes as she promised to care for him, the click of our front door closing behind me, unsure when I would open it again.

Somewhere over the Pacific, the weight of it all broke me. I pressed my face into my hands and wept quietly, torn between love and the unspoken truth that to build a better future, I had to leave part of my heart behind.

A stranger noticed, tall, white-haired, kind eyed. His voice was gentle. "Are you okay?"

I nodded, though grief sat tight in my chest. He rested a hand on my shoulder and said, "Everything will be all right."

It was such a simple phrase, but in that moment, it steadied me. It felt like grace a small sign that I wasn't completely alone. His words carried me through the rest of the flight and gave me the strength to step onto American soil believing I could endure what lay ahead.

When the plane touched down, the cold air rushed into the cabin. I remember gripping my coat tighter, unprepared for the sharp bite of winter.

Outside the terminal windows, snow flurries danced tiny white miracles that seemed to whisper, *begin again.* I didn't know it then, but that small encounter would become a metaphor for the life of every nurse: strangers crossing paths, offering comfort, reminding one another that even in uncertainty, compassion remains our compass.

In the years since, I have replayed that scene many times on nights when exhaustion pressed against my chest, on mornings when I questioned whether I had chosen the right path. Each time I returned to that memory, I found the same quiet truth: we survive by holding one another up.

That is why this book exists. It isn't only my story; it's the story of every nurse who has left the familiar for the unknown, who has faced doubt and chosen courage anyway. It's for the foreign-trained nurse who arrives with skill but no recognition, and for the new graduate who walks into a hospital with a shiny badge and a trembling heart.

It's for the parents working the night shift, the students wondering if they belong, and the mentor who still remembers what it felt like to be new.

Because no matter where we come from, every nurse starts at the same place: the intersection of fear and purpose.

I learned this quickly when I began working in an American hospital. The hallways looked nothing like the ones I trained in. The beeping monitors spoke a different rhythm, the accents carried unfamiliar words, and even the silence between conversations felt foreign. I often felt like an imposter in my own scrubs caught between what I knew and what I still needed to learn.

There were moments when I wanted to turn back, to go home, and start over. But every time, something grounded me the memory of Liam's face, the echo of that stranger's voice, the knowledge that this was bigger than my fear.

I noticed how nurses everywhere shared the same heartbeat of purpose. In the break room, I watched a colleague quietly slip half her lunch to a patient's family who hadn't eaten. In PCU, I saw a nurse stay past her shift so a dying man wouldn't be alone. None of us were heroes; we were simply people choosing compassion over convenience, again and again.

Those small acts became my teachers. They showed me that courage isn't loud; it's steady. It doesn't always look like strength; sometimes it looks like showing up even when your voice shakes.

This book is meant to be both a companion and a survival guide. The first year of nursing is hard, but it is also holy work shaping, humbling, transformative. You will question yourself, celebrate small victories, and discover strength in moments you least expect.

If I could sit with you on your first break after a long shift, I'd tell you this: the doubt you feel means you care.

The fear you carry means you understand the weight of what you've been trusted with. And the exhaustion you fight through means you're growing into the nurse you're meant to be.

My hope is that within these pages, you'll find not only stories but strategies not only lessons but reminders that you are never alone in this journey.

With the right mindset, you won't just survive your first year you'll bloom in it. You'll find purpose in the chaos, wisdom in your mistakes, and pride in every heartbeat you help steady.

This book is my way of telling you that what you feel is valid, that your beginnings matter, and that your story no matter how messy or uncertain is worth telling.

Welcome to the beginning of your story. From this point forward, the real learning begins not in classrooms or checklists, but in the hallways where courage is tested and character takes shape. This is where theory meets reality, where confidence wavers, and where you start to discover who you are as a nurse. Every shift, every patient, every challenge adds a new line to your story. And like all of us who came before you, you'll learn that the first year isn't just about surviving the work it's about becoming the kind of nurse, and the kind of person, you were always meant to be.

To understand who you are becoming, we first must look closely at who you are right now: a new graduate nurse standing at the edge of your first year. That's where our story truly begins.

— ✦ —

# CHAPTER 1

# WHO IS A NEW GRADUATE NURSE?

The rehab floor smelled of antiseptic, brewed coffee, and the faint rust of portable tanks lined along the hallway. I would later learn that every unit has its own scent 3 North sterile and cold, med-surg like lavender sanitizer, rehab like talcum and time but that first morning it was all new, all overwhelming.

The fluorescent lights hummed above, too bright against my restless heart. The tile floor gleamed like glass; my reflection blinked back in a shade of doubt I couldn't hide. My scrubs felt stiffer than courage, my shoes squeaked louder than I wanted, and the laminated ID clipped to my chest felt heavier than its plastic weight. I kept touching it, tracing my name, as though repetition could make it real: *Pia Dy, RN.*

A group of nurses passed by laughing, their steps confident, their voices blending into the rhythm of the unit's soundtrack machines beeping, phones ringing, call lights chiming. They belonged to the rhythm. I was still counting beats, trying to find where to step in.

"First day?" a voice asked.

I turned. A woman in navy scrubs, hair tied neatly, smiled at me. Her badge read Ellen, Nurse Manager.

"Yes, ma'am," I answered too quickly. My accent curled around the words; I heard it and winced.

"Don't call me ma'am," she said kindly. "That'll make me feel old. Come on, I'll show you where to sign in."

Her friendliness steadied me just enough to move my feet. We passed the nurses' station a semicircle of blinking screens, coffee cups, and Post-it Notes. Someone was laughing about a night-shift story; another was speed-typing notes with the intensity of a pianist.

"Here's your assignment," Ellen said, handing me a folded paper. "Two patients for orientation. You'll shadow Jocelyn today she's good. Don't worry, we don't expect miracles on day one."

Her voice was light, but my stomach tightened. Two patients. Two lives. Back home I had cared for entire wards, but this felt different higher stakes, higher expectations, an invisible standard I couldn't yet name.

Jocelyn appeared moments later tall and quick smiling, the kind of nurse whose calm filled the room before her words did. She extended her hand. "Welcome, Pia. We'll start slow. Promise."

We entered the first room together. The blinds were half-open; winter light spilled across a frail man attached to more wires than I could count. The monitor ticked out his heartbeat steady but fragile. He turned his head, eyes searching.

"Good morning, Mr. Smith," Jocelyn said brightly. "This is Nurse Pia, she's new with us."

His lips curved faintly. "Another angel in training, huh?"

The joke disarmed me. "Trying my best," I said softly. "Then you'll do fine." He closed his eyes again. It was such a small exchange, but it cracked something open inside me. In that moment, fear gave way to purpose. For the first time since landing in America, I felt the faintest belonging not because I was sure of myself, but because someone had trusted me enough to call me nurse.

Later, in the hallway, my hands trembled as I charted under Jocelyn's supervision. The EMR system blinked unfamiliar terms; my fingers hesitated over each dropdown menu.

"You're doing okay," Jocelyn said. "Take your time."

But time was exactly what I feared losing. Each beep, each call light, each voice over the intercom reminded me that hospitals don't wait for you to catch up. Still, I breathed, clicked, and saved one note at a time.

When my shift ended, I walked outside into the brittle air. Snow had started to fall, quiet and thin. Each flake melted on my sleeve before I could see its shape. I stood there for a long moment, exhausted yet wide awake, realizing that this was only the beginning of the long corridor between knowing and becoming.

"First day?" a voice asked.

Those two words carried more weight than I expected. It wasn't just small talk; it was initiation. Every nurse remembers the person who spoke to them first the one who broke the tension of silence when fear was loudest.

I smiled weakly, unsure if my answer sounded confident or terrified. "Yes, my first day."

"Then welcome," she said and her tone was both kind and efficient, like she had said it a thousand times before.

That's how every new nurse begins: between the comfort of knowing *something* and the unease of realizing how little that something really is. Nursing school teaches the framework: anatomy, pharmacology, pathophysiology. But no textbook can teach you how to look into the eyes of a patient in pain and not let your own voice tremble.

In class, we were told to cluster care, conserve energy, and communicate effectively. What they didn't say was that sometimes *communicate effectively* means biting your tongue, swallowing your frustration, and choosing grace instead of pride. They didn't teach us that compassion can run dry if you don't refill it, or that you'd look at the clock at 3 a.m. and realize you haven't eaten, sat down, or used the bathroom in eight hours and still, you'd have to keep going.

That's the bridge between knowing and becoming.

It isn't a quick crossing; it's built slowly, with trembling hands and uncertain steps. Each shift lays another plank. Each mistake teaches you how to hold steady when the foundation shakes.

I remember standing by a patient's bed for the first time, vital-signs machine humming, IV pump blinking orange. I knew the steps to check the line, silence the alarm, verify the medication, but my hands hesitated. *What if I get it wrong? What if the patient notices I'm not as sure as I pretend to be?*

"Go ahead," Jocelyn said gently. "You know this." I didn't realize then how important those three words were, *you know this.* She wasn't just giving permission to act; she was lending me her confidence until I found my own.

Later that evening, as we wrapped up the shift, she told me something I never forgot: "Pia, nursing isn't about memorizing protocols. It's about learning to stand still when everything else is moving."

That line stayed with me. Because every nurse learns quickly that hospitals are organized chaos. No two patients are the same, no shift unfolds the same way twice, and no amount of studying can prepare you for the first time someone grabs your hand and says, "Please don't let me die."

It's in those moments that the bridge wobbles. You look for something steady to hold on to a mentor, a routine, a prayer and you keep walking, one breath at a time.

When I went home that night, my feet ached and my mind was spinning. I replayed every small mistake: the IV line I almost kinked, the chart I forgot to sign, the awkward silence when a patient cracked a joke I didn't understand. My instinct was to focus on what went wrong, not what went right.

But that's where growth hides in reflection, not perfection.

In nursing, *becoming* isn't a moment of arrival; it's a lifelong unfolding. You don't wake up one day and feel ready. Readiness sneaks in quietly between mistakes and miracles, between tears and laughter, between who you were and who you're becoming.

There's a sacred humility that comes with realizing how much you still don't know. The best nurses I've ever met aren't the ones who act like experts; they're the ones who stay curious. They ask, *why did this patient's blood pressure drop suddenly? What else could be causing this symptom? How can I make this person's experience better next time?*

Curiosity is the bridge that keeps us learning long after orientation ends.

I wish someone had told me this sooner: it's okay not to feel ready. No one does. Even the confident nurses, the ones who seem unshakable, were once standing exactly where you are now clutching a clipboard and praying no one asks a question they can't answer.

So, if you're in that place straddling the uncertain space between student and professional know that you are right where you're supposed to be. You're not failing; you're forming. You're building that bridge one experience at a time.

And when you finally reach the other side, you'll turn around and realize something beautiful: the bridge you built isn't just for you. It's for every nurse who will follow each one crossing the same uncertain distance from *I hope I can* to *I know I can.*

For me, that bridge began long before my first day on the unit; it started the moment I crossed an actual ocean.

## Crossing Oceans

When people talk about moving abroad, they often focus on what is gained opportunity, adventure, the promise of a better life. But few talk about what is lost.

When I left the Philippines, I didn't just board a plane. I dismantled a life. Every goodbye was a quiet tearing; every step toward the gate was a choice between love and survival.

It wasn't just leaving a place; it was leaving a rhythm, a language, a version of myself that existed only in that small apartment where my son's laughter filled the evenings. On the day I left, I packed my nursing books beside a photograph of Liam in his school uniform, his smile wide and certain. He didn't understand the magnitude of what was happening. "See you soon, Mom," he said, not knowing that *soon* would mean years.

The flight to America was long enough to relive an entire life. I remember the cabin lights dimmed, passengers asleep, and me staring out the small oval window into a sky that had no borders. Somewhere below was the ocean that divided us wide, silent, endless.

People say distance makes the heart grow fonder. In truth, distance makes the heart grow disciplined. It teaches you to hold love differently not with your arms, but with your endurance.

When I arrived in New Jersey, the air was sharp and cold. The airport buzzed with voices tumbling over one another accents, laughter, commands. Everything felt too fast, too loud. Even the carts moved differently.

An agency representative greeted me with a sign bearing my name. "Welcome, Nurse Pia," he said. His words were kind but rehearsed. I was one of hundreds of nurses being ushered into a new life. To them, I was a file, a contract, a placement. To me, this was a once-in-a-lifetime leap of faith.

That night in the shared staff housing, I sat on the narrow bed, surrounded by unpacked luggage and dim light, listening to the unfamiliar hum of a radiator. The air smelled faintly of old wood and loneliness. I taped Liam's picture beside my pillow and whispered a promise: *One day, I'll make this worth it.*

The first weeks were a blur of paperwork, orientations, and policy training. My mouth grew tired from smiling. My ears strained to keep up with rapid English, idioms I had never heard, and the clipped tone of efficiency that American healthcare thrives on.

During the first hospital orientation, the instructor's voice echoed through the auditorium: "We expect our nurses to practice autonomy, critical thinking, and time management."

I scribbled notes furiously, pretending to understand. *Autonomy* sounded empowering but also isolating. In the Philippines, nursing was teamwork to the bone. We leaned on each other, shared meals, and laughed through chaos. Here, I was on my own one nurse, one assignment, one expectation: perform flawlessly.

At lunch, a few of us foreign nurses huddled in the corner of the cafeteria, clutching our sandwiches like lifelines. There was Joy from Cebu, who, like me, had never seen snow before, and Rafi from Mumbai, who kept checking his phone for messages from home. We laughed nervously, mixing English and our native tongues, trading stories of visa struggles and missing family birthdays.

Despite our differences, we were united by the same silent truth: we had crossed oceans not because we wanted to leave home, but because home had run out of options.

The first time someone commented on my accent, I froze. "Wow, you speak English really well," they said, surprised. It was meant as a compliment, but it landed like a reminder: *you are other.*

Another time, a coworker joked, "You're lucky. You're from a tropical country, right? Bet this snow feels like punishment."

I smiled politely, the way many immigrants do when grace feels safer than confrontation. But inside, something shifted. I realized that assimilation wasn't just about language or skill, it was about invisibility. To belong, I would have to learn how to shrink parts of myself.

It was in those quiet moments of shrinking that I began to understand belonging in a deeper way not as disappearance, but as transformation. Every misunderstanding became an invitation to grow more fluent in empathy.

I started to see my difference not as a liability but as strength. My accent carried the echo of resilience; my hands carried years of experience. I began to understand that cultural humility flows both ways. Yes, I had to adapt, but they could also learn from me from my empathy, my patience, my ability to care even when words stumbled.

Humor became my translator. When I didn't understand an idiom, I asked with a laugh. That broke the ice more times than I can count. Slowly, the walls softened.

There were still moments of isolation. Nights when I'd walk home from the facility under a navy sky, the city lights flickering like distant promises. The world was asleep, but my mind was loud replaying every interaction, every mispronounced word, every reminder that I was a guest in someone else's country.

And yet, amid the loneliness, small miracles bloomed.

A patient's daughter once told me, "You remind me of my mom soft-spoken but strong."

A charge nurse noticed my careful notes and said, "You're thorough. I like that."

A physician thanked me for catching a medication error before it reached the patient.

Each moment stitched another thread of belonging. Not validation but quiet recognition.

Being a foreign-trained nurse meant living in translation translating not just language, but culture, emotion, and self. It meant learning when to speak and when silence said enough. It meant turning homesickness into fuel and finding joy in the smallest connections: a patient calling me *dear*, a coworker offering to split her lunch, a phone call from home that began with "We're proud of you."

Years later, when I teach new nurses, I tell them: "Crossing oceans isn't just about geography. Every nurse crosses one between who they were and who they're becoming."

The geography of growth looks different for everyone, but the feeling is the same: the vertigo of starting over, the ache of missing what's familiar, the slow dawning of strength you didn't know you had.

If I could go back to that first night in staff housing, I'd tell the woman staring at Liam's photo that she's not losing herself, she's expanding. That the distance she feels now will one day become her greatest empathy. That the ocean between where she came from and where she stands is not a divide; it's a bridge.

And on that bridge, she will find herself becoming not just a nurse, but a citizen of compassion. That bridge carried me straight into the everyday reality of my new life: a rehabilitation facility that would quietly become my first real classroom.

## Learning the Language of Care

The first day I walked into the rehabilitation facility, it didn't look anything like the hospitals I'd seen on television or the ones where I'd trained back home. There were no fast-moving trauma teams, no dramatic codes, no blaring alarms. Instead, the air was thick with antiseptic and the faint scent of lotion. Wheelchairs rolled slowly down wide corridors. The rhythm here wasn't crisis, it was endurance.

When someone said, "I'm bushed," it took me weeks to realize they meant "I'm overwhelmed." When a nurse asked me to "hang a banana bag," I looked around for a rope before realizing she meant an IV medication. Every phrase was a puzzle, every instruction a new dialect of nursing that I had to decode in real time.

At first, my hands worked faster than my understanding. I relied on instinct, repetition, and observation. I memorized not only the tasks but the rhythm: the way experienced nurses anticipated call lights, the way they multitasked without panic, the way they spoke to families in voices that were both calm and commanding.

There was a quiet choreography to care that no textbook had ever mentioned. Nurses moved around one another like dancers who'd learned the same steps years ago. I tried to mimic them pushing stretchers, answering phones, adjusting IV pumps, all while pretending I wasn't terrified.

But every evening, when I clocked out, I carried questions home like uncharted maps. *Did I say the right thing to that patient? Did I wash my hands enough? Did they notice my accent when I was giving report?*

Over time, I realized that learning the language of care wasn't just about speaking English fluently, it was about learning the emotional grammar of nursing.

It was learning how silence can comfort more than words. How a gentle nod can say *I see you.* How to read the subtle tension in a patient's face before pain shows up in their vitals.

One afternoon, I met Mr. Cooper, a stroke survivor with halting speech and eyes that darted between hope and frustration. Communication between us was clumsy at first. He would point, I would guess, we'd both laugh when I got it wrong.

Then one day, while helping him stand for physical therapy, I said softly, "I know it's hard, but we'll do this together."

He squeezed my hand with surprising strength and whispered, "You understand."

It was just two words, but they bridged an entire ocean. That moment taught me that empathy is a universal language spoken not with words, but with presence.

Still, not every moment was tender. There were times when I made small mistakes enough to bruise my confidence. I once forgot to sign a vital-signs sheet; another time I documented on the wrong chart. Nothing catastrophic, but enough to make me question whether I belonged.

I remember sitting in the supply room once, staring at the floor tiles as tears stung my eyes. The room was empty except for the low hum of the medication refrigerator. I whispered a prayer not for strength, but for clarity: *Am I meant for this?*

Minutes later, another nurse walked in Angela, one of the night-shift regulars. She didn't say anything at first, just handed me a paper towel to wipe my eyes. Then she said, "You'll be fine, Pia. We've all been there. You're learning. That's what counts."

Those words were simple but sacred. In that small act of kindness, I learned that mentorship doesn't always look formal; it often appears as a colleague handing you grace when you can't give it to yourself.

Every shift after that felt a little lighter. I began to ask more questions, to take notes during report, to stay a few minutes after shift to review my charts. Slowly, confidence became less of a feeling and more of a habit.

The rehabilitation unit became my classroom. The patients were my teachers, the nurses, my translators. I learned that healing is never one-directional, it flows both ways. As much as I helped patients recover their strength, they helped me recover my courage.

There was Mrs. Daniels, who made me promise to visit her garden when she got discharged. There was Raymond, who taught me that laughter could lower blood pressure faster than any pill. And there was quiet Mr. Singh, who, before being discharged, told me in a soft accent, "You remind me of my daughter. Keep helping people."

I kept those words like a talisman.

By the end of my first year, the language of care had become second nature. I could sense what a patient needed before they spoke. I could interpret the difference between a pain grimace and an anxious frown. I could walk into a room and feel its emotional temperature change before the monitors caught up.

That's when I realized that nursing was never about mastering tasks, it was about mastering connection.

To learn the language of care, you must listen beyond words. You must read gestures, feel silences, and understand that healing often begins in the spaces where language fails.

And just like that, I began to feel fluent, not in English, but in compassion. But even as compassion became my new fluency, the weight of responsibility was still waiting to test everything I thought I'd learned.

## Reality Shock

The first year of nursing is often called *reality shock.* It's the moment when the safety net of school gives way to the full weight of responsibility. You leave the structure of classrooms for the chaos of hospital life. Real people. Real pain. Real consequences.

I had read about this transition, how it crushes some and strengthens others, but nothing could prepare me for the way it would shake me to my core.

There's a moment every nurse remembers: the first time you realize someone's life depends on your judgment, your timing, your hands. Mine came late on a double shift.

The lights of the rehab unit had dimmed, and most patients were asleep. The quiet hum of oxygen machines filled the air, broken only by the occasional shuffle of slippers. I was checking on Mr. Patel, a patient recovering from a complicated stroke, when I noticed his breathing change shallow, uneven. His skin had taken on that faint gray tint I had only seen in textbooks.

My heart began to race. My hands trembled slightly as I reached for the call button. "Jocelyn," I whispered to my preceptor, "Can you come here?"

When she arrived, she took one look and said, "Call the rapid response."

Everything that happened next blurred into instinct. I called out vitals, handed equipment, checked IV access. My training surfaced, but fear fought to drown it out. As the code team arrived, I stepped back, heart pounding. They worked with precision, calling out orders in quick succession. And then, just as suddenly as it began, it was over. Mr. Patel was stabilized.

When the team left, I stood there frozen. Jocelyn turned to me and said quietly, "You did good."

But I didn't feel good. I felt cracked open. The adrenaline had masked it in the moment, but now all I could feel was the weight of it, the awareness that a single missed cue could have changed everything.

That night, I went home, dropped my bag on the floor, and cried until the edges of the room blurred. The tears weren't just for fear or exhaustion; they were for the distance from home, for the grief I still carried, for the question that haunted me: *Am I strong enough for this?*

Reality shock isn't just about stress. It's about identity. It forces you to confront who you thought you were and who you are under pressure.

Some mornings, I would wake up still tired, stare at my reflection, and whisper, "You can do this." I'd remind myself of every patient who'd smiled, every colleague who'd encouraged me, every small victory that proved I was growing.

But there were also mornings I wanted to quit.

I remember once being so overwhelmed that I forgot to eat my entire twelve-hour shift. By 5 p.m., my head was throbbing and my charting lagged. A nurse passing by said, "You're behind again, Pia." Her tone wasn't cruel, just factual but it hit me like a verdict.

That evening, I sat in my car long after my shift ended, gripping the steering wheel, staring at my reflection in the rearview mirror. I didn't recognize the woman looking back at me her eyes tired, her spirit frayed, her confidence somewhere back on the unit floor.

And then, in that silence, I heard my own voice say what I tell my students now: *You don't have to be perfect to belong here. You just must keep showing up.*

So, I did.

Every day I showed up. I listened more, asked questions without shame, and learned to forgive myself faster.

There were days when chaos tested my patience when alarms screamed, families shouted, and physicians barked orders but there were also moments of grace that kept me anchored. A patient who whispered, "Thank you for not rushing me." A coworker sliding a cup of coffee across the desk after a difficult shift. A supervisor saying quietly, "You handled that beautifully."

Nursing has a way of breaking you open and then rebuilding you stronger, layer by layer. The pressure doesn't just forge skill; it refines compassion.

Reality shock taught me something no textbook ever could. Resilience doesn't mean you don't feel overwhelmed, it means you keep standing even when you do.

As weeks turned into months, I began to recognize myself again not the uncertain nurse from my first day, but someone steadier, someone who could be trusted. I no longer trembled when the charge nurse said, "You've got the tough patient today." I no longer doubted whether I belonged.

I learned that strength in nursing isn't loud or visible. It's quiet. It's the kind of strength that shows up in the middle of the night when you're holding a patient's hand, or in the calm voice you use when everyone else is panicking.

By the end of that first year, I realized something profound: survival itself is a success.

If my patients made it safely through my shift, if their families left reassured, if my coworkers could rely on me that was victory enough.

Confidence, I discovered, doesn't come in a single leap. It's layered slowly shift after shift, lesson after mistake, small triumph after small triumph. Every patient became a teacher: how to listen beyond words, how to advocate firmly but kindly, how to stay gentle when the world isn't.

That's the paradox of nursing: it both hardens and softens you. It demands precision but rewards compassion. It exposes your flaws but reveals your strength. And it never truly stops teaching.

In that constant classroom of reality, the people who stood beside me became some of my most powerful teachers.

## Finding My Mentors

One of my greatest teachers was not a physician but a Haitian nurse named Marie. She saw me floundering before I realized it myself. There was something about her steady, unhurried, unbothered by the chaos around her. While others barked orders or sighed in frustration, Marie seemed to move through the day with a rhythm I could only admire.

"Stay calm, stay organized, keep going," she would say. It was her mantra, and eventually, it became mine.

Marie's presence anchored me in ways I didn't expect. She corrected without condescension and celebrated small wins others might not notice. "Your charting's cleaner today," she'd point out. Or "Good catch on that med timing." Those words mattered more than she knew.

There was a day I nearly quit. It was a Sunday double shift the kind that blurs one day into another. The unit was short-staffed, and I had more patients than I could safely manage. One of them, a postoperative man with uncontrolled pain kept pressing the call bell every few minutes. I was behind on meds, documentation, and discharges. My head was pounding, my confidence unraveling by the minute.

When I finally reached his room, I could feel the weight of frustration in his glare. "You nurses don't care," he said bitterly. "You leave people suffering."

The words sliced deep. I apologized softly, adjusted his position, and administered the delayed medication. My hands trembled slightly as I flushed the IV line. I wanted to explain, to make him see that I was doing my best, but I also knew he didn't need an explanation. He needed relief.

When I stepped out, Marie was waiting near the med cart. She looked at me for a long moment before saying, "You can cry later. Right now, finish strong."

Her voice wasn't unkind. It was truth, wrapped in love.

We sat together during the short break that followed. She shared a story from her own first year, a shift when she was so overwhelmed she dropped a full medication tray on the floor and had to start over from scratch. "I wanted to walk out that day," she said. "But a nurse told me, 'You're not failing, you're learning under pressure.' And here I am, still learning, still standing."

That conversation changed how I saw struggle.

I realized that mentorship isn't about rescuing someone; it's about reminding them of their strength.

Through Marie, I learned that experience is meant to be shared, not hoarded. The best nurses aren't those who know everything, but those who remember what it felt like not to.

She taught me small, practical things no manual ever covered how to chart as I go, how to prioritize when everything feels urgent, how to keep an extra pair of gloves in my pocket because "you never know."

But she also taught me invisible skills: the art of staying kind when I'm exhausted, the discipline of taking a breath before reacting, the humility of saying *thank you* even when I've been corrected.

Over time, I realized that mentorship is a quiet form of legacy. It's how wisdom travels from one nurse to another through whispered advice at the bedside, through a gentle correction in the charting room, through a look that says, *you've got this.*

Eventually, Marie introduced me to others who became my circle of mentors:

- Maria, the night-shift RN who taught me the value of humor in chaos.
- Nancy, the wound-care specialist who showed me that precision is compassion.
- Wanda, the soft-spoken CNA who modeled patience that could calm even the angriest patient.

They weren't just colleagues; they were lifelines. Each left fingerprints on my practice.

Sometimes, mentorship came from people I barely knew. A respiratory therapist once handed me a cup of water during a code and said, "Breathe, nurse. You're part of the team now." That single sentence stitched my frayed nerves back together.

Looking back, I see now that mentorship is the heartbeat of nursing. Without it, the profession would fracture under its own weight. With it, we not only survive, but we also multiply strength.

To this day, when I mentor new nurses, I repeat Marie's words: "Stay calm, stay organized, keep going." And I add my own: "Ask questions. Be humble. Say thank you twice as often as you complain."

Because somewhere out there, another new nurse is standing exactly where I once stood unsure, exhausted, trembling and waiting for someone to remind her she can do this.

That's how we pay it forward. That's how the lineage of compassion continues. Their belief in me did more than get me through hard shifts; it quietly reshaped who I was becoming at the bedside.

## Becoming

The first time I handled an emergency alone, my hands shook so badly I almost dropped the blood-pressure cuff. The patient's alarms blared like sirens in my chest, and for a split second the room shrank around me. Then, like an echo, I heard Marie's voice in my mind: *Stay calm. Stay organized. Keep going.*

I inhaled, steadied my hands, and began to move. Assess first. Call for help. Reassure the patient. My training rose to the surface like a life raft. The monitors began to normalize, and so did my breathing. When the charge nurse walked in moments later, she found not a frantic new nurse, but a focused one.

When it was over, I leaned against the wall, sweat cooling on my forehead. Relief flooded me not because I had been flawless, but because I had acted. I hadn't frozen, I hadn't faltered, and for the first time, I saw a glimpse of the nurse I was becoming.

From that day on, something subtle but permanent shifted inside me. I stopped measuring myself against the nurses who seemed perfect. Instead, I started measuring against who I was yesterday. Every small victory remembering a complex med schedule, catching an early sign of infection, advocating for a patient who couldn't became a milestone.

Confidence, I discovered, wasn't a single moment of triumph. It was built from repetition, patience, and forgiveness. It was in the way I began to walk down the hallway, shoulders back, steps measured, eyes scanning the environment with purpose. My badge no longer felt borrowed; it felt earned.

Soon, other nurses started coming to me with small questions. "Hey, Pia, how do you chart wound care again?" or "Can you help me with this discharge?" The first time it happened, I almost laughed, *me,* the one who used to Google every abbreviation? But I realized mentorship isn't just for those with decades of experience; it's for anyone willing to lift someone else while still climbing.

There were still hard days when the patient load was impossible, when families took their pain out on me, when grief sat heavy after a loss I couldn't prevent. But there were also moments of quiet grace that stitched the hard days together:

- A patient whispering, "You made me feel safe."
- A doctor thanking me for noticing a subtle change that prevented a fall.

- A coworker sliding a granola bar into my pocket after a 13-hour shift.

These were the currencies of resilience.

Nursing began to teach me about balance that you can be exhausted and still gentle, that you can feel fear and still act bravely, that you can make mistakes and still be worthy of trust.

I started keeping a small notebook in my scrub pocket. After each shift, I'd jot down one thing I did well. It wasn't about pride; it was about proof. Proof that I was growing, that my efforts mattered even when no one noticed. On bad days, those notes reminded me that progress is cumulative you just can't always see it in the moment.

One afternoon, after a particularly complex dressing change, Marie smiled and said, "See? You're not the new nurse anymore."

I laughed, shaking my head. "I still feel new most days."

"Good," she said. "That's how you stay teachable."

Her words stayed with me. Being new, I realized, isn't just about time; it's about curiosity. The best nurses never stop being students.

As the months passed, I found a rhythm one that belonged to me. I learned when to speak and when to listen, when to rush and when to pause, when to hold a patient's hand and when to let go. I learned that leadership doesn't always wear a title; sometimes it's as simple as setting the tone for the shift calm, kind, steady.

The fear that once paralyzed me became the quiet fuel that kept me sharp. Every challenge turned into a chance to prove that I could adapt, grow, and stand tall even under pressure.

And perhaps most importantly, I began to see nursing not as a job, but as a mirror. Every interaction reflected something about who I was my patience, my values, my capacity for grace. The more I cared for others, the more I understood myself.

One winter morning, as I was leaving after a night shift, I caught my reflection in the glass doors of the hospital. My hair was messy under my cap, my eyes tired, but there was a calm in my face I hadn't seen before. Behind me, the monitors beeped faintly, and in that sound, I heard the rhythm of belonging.

I smiled. Not because I had arrived, but because I was no longer afraid of where I was going.

That's when I finally understood what every seasoned nurse tries to tell the new ones:

You don't wake up one day and become a nurse.

You build her shift by shift, patient by patient, mistake by mistake until one day you look up and realize she's been inside you all along. As you read this chapter, I don't want you to just follow my story; I want you to begin noticing your own.

## Reflections

1. When did you last doubt yourself, and how did you move through it?
2. Doubt often visits when you care deeply. Write about a moment when uncertainty crept in perhaps during a difficult shift or when you felt unseen and then describe what helped you

move forward. Was it a patient's gratitude? A mentor's reassurance? Or your own decision to keep showing up despite the fear? Every time you reflect on how you pushed through, you collect evidence of your strength.

3. What moments big or small remind you why you chose nursing?
4. Remember the sound of laughter after pain eases, the gratitude in a patient's eyes, the warmth of teamwork in crisis. Nursing is full of hidden rewards, often tucked inside ordinary days. List a few of those moments here. Let them anchor you when fatigue and doubt cloud your purpose.
5. Who has been your "Marie," the person whose belief in you steadied your steps?
6. Write their name. Recall what they said, how they helped you breathe easier, how they modeled grace under pressure. Gratitude transforms memory into fuel; acknowledging your mentors reminds you that you are never truly alone in this journey.

*Take time to write your answers. Reflection turns experience into wisdom. What feels like struggle today will one day become part of your strength story.*

And while reflection shapes your inner strength, there are also concrete habits that can help you make it through the hardest days.

## Survival Tips

- **Breathe before you act.**
  A calm nurse is a safe nurse. When chaos erupts, your breath is your first assessment tool. It grounds your body and clears your thinking. One deep breath can be the difference between reacting and responding.
- **Find mentors.**
  Wisdom shared is strength multiplied. Seek nurses who correct with kindness and lead by example. And when you're ready, become that person for someone else. Mentorship is the invisible thread that keeps nursing connected through generations.
- **Keep learning.**
  Every patient is a teacher in disguise. Read, observe, ask *why.* Curiosity keeps your practice alive. The moment you stop learning; you stop growing and growth is what transforms work into calling.
- **Protect your rest.**
  Fatigue distorts judgment; self-care is patient care. Rest is not indulgence it's maintenance. Learn to rest without guilt, to say *no* when your body says *enough.*
- **Celebrate progress.**
  Each small improvement builds confidence. Write down your wins, however tiny: a well-timed IV, a grateful smile, a shift with fewer errors. Success in nursing isn't measured in perfection; it's measured in persistence.

- **Document your wins.**
  Keep a small notebook or a note on your phone. On difficult days, reread it. It's easy to forget how far you've come when you're still walking uphill.

All these practices are small on their own, but together they create a foundation you can stand on when the year feels heavier than you imagined.

## Closing Thoughts

The first year of nursing will test your patience, stamina, and heart and it will build you. You may feel unprepared and small, but every step you take, every patient you help, and every tear you wipe away teaches you what it truly means to serve.

There will be nights when exhaustion feels heavier than purpose. There will be mornings when doubt lingers longer than sunlight. But remember this: each shift you complete, each challenge you overcome, is evidence that you are becoming stronger, wiser, more compassionate.

You'll look back and realize you were never an imposter. You were a nurse in formation being shaped by every experience, molded by every lesson, and strengthened by every person who crossed your path.

Someday, a new nurse will stand where you once stood unsure, anxious, eager to belong. You'll see yourself in their trembling hands and hopeful eyes. When that moment comes, smile. You've come full circle. You've become the mentor you once needed.

## 🖉 Notes

*(Use this space to write your reflections, lessons learned, or next-shift intentions.)*

______________________________________________

______________________________________________

______________________________________________

______________________________________________

______________________________________________

______________________________________________

Every nurse remembers the early timeline that shapes them the first day, the first week, the first month when everything still feels new and impossibly big.

# CHAPTER 2

# YOUR FIRST DAY, FIRST WEEK, FIRST MONTH

*"At first, everything feels impossible until one day, it feels familiar." — Unknown*

Leaving the slower rhythm of the rehabilitation facility behind, I walked through the doors of my first hospital assignment in the United States with my heart pounding. I had prayed for this moment and promised I would rise to the challenge, but nothing could have fully prepared me for what awaited on the other side of those glass doors.

The step-down unit was alive with motion. Call bells rang in quick succession, monitors beeped in overlapping patterns, and the air seemed to pulse with urgency. The lights felt harsher, the voices sharper, the pace faster than anything I had ever known. I gripped my folded assignment sheet so tightly my fingers ached, hoping no one could see how nervous I was.

Beside me stood my preceptor, Valsa, a senior nurse with years of experience and a quiet authority that filled the hallway. Thin gold bangles jingled softly at her wrist a sound that would become oddly comforting as the days unfolded. Her accent carried a gentle lilt, but what stood out most was her tone warm, motherly, yet firm when needed. From the first moment, she made me feel safe to learn, as if her calm would hold me steady while I found my footing. Still, no amount of reassurance could soften the shock of that very first shift.

## Day One — Baptism by Beeping

The unit wasted no time testing me.

An IV pump blared *INFUSION COMPLETE.* I froze for a heartbeat, my mind scrambling.

"Pia, that's yours," Valsa said calmly. "Go ahead and flush and remember to chart it."

Her reassurance steadied me, but anxiety still coiled in my stomach. This wasn't a simulation lab; this was a living human being my patient, my responsibility. My hands moved with cautious precision even as my thoughts raced. Back home I was used to gravity drips and manual calculations. Here, everything was sleek, electronic, and demanding. Every alarm was a language I had yet to learn.

Even the smallest differences reminded me how far I was from home. When Valsa asked if I had given *Robitussin*, her pronunciation "ROH-bi-tuh-sin" felt strange to my ear. In the Philippines we said "ROH-bi-TOO-sin." That tiny detail made me suddenly aware of how foreign I must have sounded. Under my breath I practiced until the new rhythm rolled naturally off my tongue. I wanted my patients to hear confidence, not distance.

By midday, exhaustion pressed down like a heavy blanket. I had answered call bells, adjusted IV fluids, fielded family questions, and charted more than I thought possible. Each task took twice as long as it should have. The electronic record seemed endless, each click a reminder of the responsibility I carried.

At one point, Valsa caught me staring at the screen, my face tight with worry. She rested a hand on my shoulder, bangles chiming softly.

"Everyone feels this way on their first day," she said. "Breathe. You're doing well."

Those words became a lifeline proof that even seasoned nurses once stood where I stood.

When the shift finally ended, I walked to my car in silence. The evening air was cool and still. Beneath the exhaustion sat a quiet pride: I had made it through not flawlessly, but faithfully.

That night, I wrote a single line in my notebook:

*Survived my first shift. Someday, I'll thrive through one.*

What I didn't realize then was that surviving one day was only the beginning; soon the days would blur into a week that stretched me even further.

## Week One — Controlled Chaos

The first week felt like being dropped onto a treadmill that never slowed.

Days began before sunrise and ended long after dark. I shadowed Valsa closely, following her through the maze of hallways and patient rooms, trying to mimic her composure. She moved with a rhythm that was almost musical steady, deliberate, purposeful.

I stumbled often, always a step behind. My brain sheet became a collage of arrows, abbreviations, and reminders scribbled in frantic handwriting. But confusion, I learned, wasn't failure; it was part of the process.

Time management became my steepest hill. One patient needed pain medication, another required discharge teaching, and a new admission waited at the door.

"What comes first?" I asked, breathless.

"Safety and priority, Pia," Valsa reminded me. "Handle what can't wait. Everything else follows."

It sounded simple. Living it amid alarms and demands was not. I learned to pause, assess, and act with purpose to balance what was urgent with what was important.

Charting was another mountain. The electronic record had dozens of tabs, and I worried a wrong click could lead to a dangerous omission. More than once, I asked Valsa where something belonged. She never lost patience.

"You'll get faster," she said. "Remember: the patient is the priority. The chart is the story. Don't let the screen take your eyes off the person."

Slowly, documentation became less of a task and more of a conversation a way to narrate the patient's journey.

I made mistakes, too. Once, I nearly signed off a medication without scanning. The machine beeped angrily; my face burned.

"This is why we scan," Valsa said softly. "It protects the patient and you."

Her corrections were firm but never cruel. Compassionate accountability made me want to improve, not hide.

By week's end, I realized that every delay, error, and moment of panic was quietly reshaping me. I was starting to think like a nurse anticipating, prioritizing, and finding steadiness amid chaos.

In my notes that week, I wrote:

*Confidence grows in the cracks between mistakes and mentorship.*

As the weeks passed, those small cracks of learning began to form the outline of something steadier a rhythm I could finally recognize.

## Month One — Finding Rhythm

The emotional toll was heavy. More than once, I slipped into the supply room just to breathe and blink away tears. Yet small victories appeared like constellations: locating supplies without help, introducing myself to families with confidence, recognizing accents that once confused me. Each success stitched another thread of belonging.

By the end of that first month, the hospital no longer felt like a labyrinth. The alarms became background music. Door codes rolled off my fingers. Routines emerged like constellations from chaos.

Mornings brimmed with medication passes and rounds. Afternoons brought discharges and admissions. Evenings hummed with the quiet tension of handoff reports.

Then came the day Valsa handed me my own assignment.

"This one is yours," she said. "I'll be nearby if you need me."

My heart leapt, but I nodded. It was time.

Mid-shift, a patient clutched his chest, grimacing. Instinct took over. I checked vitals, called the physician, and prepared for a possible rapid response. My hands trembled, but my voice stayed steady. All the repetition, the sleepless nights, the whispered prayers they converged in that moment.

When the patient stabilized, Valsa touched my arm.

"You kept him safe. That is what matters."

Her words sank deep. I trusted what I knew. The nurse I was becoming had arrived.

Not every day ended in triumph. One evening I forgot to reassess pain after giving a narcotic, a small oversight with serious implications. Valsa's tone was gentle but firm: "Documentation protects both of you. Never skip it."

Embarrassment burned, but I carried that lesson forward. Accountability isn't punishment; it's protection.

By month's end, I could anticipate the rhythm of the floor the times to eat quickly, to prepare ahead, and to pause long enough to breathe. The fear that once paralyzed me had turned into respect for the craft and the responsibility it carried.

If I could speak to the version of myself from that first day, I'd say: Yes, it will feel overwhelming.

Yes, you will doubt yourself. But by the end of the week, you'll see progress. By the end of the month, you'll see yourself differently.

Being overwhelmed isn't weakness; it's growth. Every nurse you admire has felt this same uncertainty. The hospital doesn't expect perfection it expects presence, compassion, and a willingness to learn. Mentors like Valsa are the quiet architects of our confidence: firm when you need direction, motherly when you need care, and wise enough to step back when it's your turn to stand alone.

Nursing isn't something you master; it's something you grow into. Slowly. Steadily. Beautifully. Now, I want you to pause and notice your own beginnings.

## Reflections

1. What emotions do you remember most from your first week fear, pride, or a mix of both?
2. Write freely. Fear means you're stretching; pride means you're recognizing progress. Both are part of growth.
3. Who are the "Valsas" in your journey those who balance correction with compassion?
4. List their names. Gratitude written down becomes a form of mentorship returned.
5. How can you pass that same grace to someone newer than you?
6. Imagine what words you needed to hear then. Offer those words now.

*Write your answers. Your growth deserves to be witnessed especially by you.* Alongside reflection, you'll also need simple, steady habits to carry you through those first disorienting weeks.

## Survival Tips

- **Listen twice, act once.**
  Composure keeps patients safe and prevents regret.
- **Document early, document accurately.**
  Memory fades faster than you think.
- **Find a rhythm, not perfection.**
  Nursing is flow, not formula.
- **Ask for feedback.**
  It's the quickest way to grow confidence and humility together.
- **Take small breaks.**
  Even a deep breath in the supply room counts as self-care.
- **End every shift with reflection.**
  Ask: *What went well? What can I do better tomorrow?*

Taken together, these small practices quietly shape the way you move through those early days.

## Closing Thoughts

Your first day, first week, and first month will test you in ways you never imagined but they'll also reveal how capable you truly are. Patterns will emerge, victories will accumulate, and confidence will grow with time. Being overwhelmed is proof you're learning.

Trust the process. Lean on your mentors. Remember that growth never looks graceful while it's happening, but every stumble is choreography for the nurse you're becoming.

By the end of your first month, you won't just recognize the hospital's rhythm you'll recognize your own. Once you can feel that rhythm, the next step is learning how to stand steadily inside it.

## Notes

*(Use this space to jot your reflections or affirmations for your next shift.)*

—✦—

# CHAPTER 3

# Finding Your Footing

*"You don't rise to the level of your goals; you fall to the level of your systems." — James Clear*

By the end of my first month on the step-down unit, something shifted inside me. The hospital no longer felt like a maze I would never escape. The sounds of call bells, alarms, and hurried footsteps became the rhythm of my day. The layout of the supply rooms, the codes to locked doors, even the sequence of tasks began to feel familiar. What once overwhelmed me now felt like a pattern I could anticipate. I wasn't fast or flawless yet, but I was no longer lost. I was finding my footing.

There is a strange comfort in realizing that chaos can become predictable. The beeping monitors that once made my heart race faded into background noise. I could tell, by tone alone, which alarm came from which room. I began to understand that mastery in nursing isn't about eliminating noise; it's about learning how to hear through it.

Some mornings still started with doubt. I'd park my car in the same corner of the lot, hands gripping the steering wheel for a few seconds longer than necessary, whispering a quiet prayer. *Lord, help me keep them safe today. Help me not miss anything.* It became my quiet ritual a grounding moment before the doors slid open and the hum of the hospital swallowed me whole.

Once inside, the fluorescent lights cast their familiar glow, bouncing off polished floors and stainless-steel carts. The scent of disinfectant mixed with freshly brewed coffee drifted down the hall. I could hear laughter from the break room, the squeak of rubber soles, the hum of machines that never slept. This was my world now fast, relentless, alive.

When I first started, these same sights and sounds felt intimidating. Now they felt like the pulse of something bigger than me, a living organism of care and coordination. Every nurse, physician, and technician moved in rhythm, weaving an invisible choreography of compassion and urgency. I wasn't yet a solo dancer in that rhythm, but I was finally moving with it.

The first sign of belonging, I realized, is when you stop counting hours and start counting wins not perfect outcomes, but moments of presence. The time you caught a near miss, reassured a frightened family, or remembered a small detail that made someone's day easier. Nursing wasn't about perfection; it was about pattern recognition both in patients and in yourself.

I noticed the shift in my own internal tempo. My movements, once halting and uncertain, became steadier. I learned where every supply lived, which physician preferred concise updates versus long ones, which coworkers would stay calm during chaos. Familiarity doesn't erase fear, but it makes room for focus. I was no longer trying to survive the shift; I was starting to *live* it.

Part of that confidence came from recognizing the unit's daily flow. Mornings were always the most demanding medications due, physicians rounding, families seeking answers all at once. The energy in the halls was like a current pulling you forward, ready or not. The scent of coffee drifted from the break room, mingling with disinfectant and the faint metallic tang of saline.

Afternoons were slightly less frantic but carried their own pressure. Discharges had to be completed, admissions arrived, and the phone never stopped. Sunlight through the narrow window by the nurses' station reminded me of the world outside, yet there was satisfaction in keeping pace with the rhythm inside.

Evenings quieted the pace but not the responsibility. It was the time to tie up loose ends, hand off to the next shift, and make sure no detail was missed. Sometimes that meant double-checking a blood sugar at the last minute or rushing to print a discharge summary before night shift arrived. Every transition was a handoff of trust.

Slowly, I recognized these rhythms and used them to pace myself to anticipate what was coming rather than react after the fact. My steps steadied, my breathing calmed. The shift no longer controlled me. I had learned to flow with it.

One night, standing near the window overlooking the parking lot, I caught my reflection in the glass-tired eyes, messy ponytail, coffee-stained badge and for the first time, I smiled. Not because I had mastered everything, but because I was *still here.* The hospital hadn't swallowed me whole; I was becoming part of it.

Finding your footing, I learned, isn't about confidence arriving all at once. It's about stringing together a thousand small moments of not giving up and realizing one day that you're standing taller than before. What once felt like survival slowly began to feel like belonging. Each chaotic moment began to reveal its own rhythm, and I realized that confidence is not built in leaps, but in steady, faithful steps.

To turn those faithful steps into something I could rely on, I had to start building systems that would hold me up on the hard days.

## Building Systems That Keep You Steady

Confidence, I learned, isn't just a feeling that comes with time, it's a *structure* you build brick by brick. It's the checklist you refine, the habits you repeat, the rhythm you protect when everything else feels uncertain.

Early in my career, I thought confidence meant "knowing everything." But after a few near-misses, I realized that true steadiness comes from creating *systems* that protect you when fatigue and stress threaten to undo your focus. It's not willpower it's architecture.

When the floor felt chaotic, these systems became my anchors. The first anchor was a simple ritual that changed the way every day began.

## My 3–2–1 Start-of-Shift Ritual

Before each shift, I gave myself five quiet minutes at the computer, even when everyone else rushed to grab vitals or prep meds. That short pause was my mental "pre-flight check."

**3 minutes** to skim overnight events and labs for each patient. I'd jot quick notes, a hemoglobin trending down, a potassium correction, a new order tucked into the chart. Those three minutes often prevented hours of confusion later.

**2 priorities** I had to accomplish before 10 a.m. They were always safety-based: a lab draw, an antibiotic, a dressing change that couldn't wait. These became my compass when interruptions flooded in.

**1 connection** I promised to make with each patient a moment beyond the checklist. Maybe asking how they slept, complimenting their progress, or simply holding their hand. I realized that even on the busiest days, patients remember compassion long after they forget your efficiency.

One morning, after a night of restless sleep, I nearly skipped the ritual. "I'll catch up later," I told myself. By 9:00 a.m., my mind was already spinning. Orders were flying in, new labs, a transport request. I was losing track until I stopped, closed my eyes for ten seconds, and restarted my 3–2–1.

By 10 a.m., both antibiotics were hung, the potassium recheck completed, and a patient smiled when I asked about his favorite hometown meal. That pause didn't slow me down; it centered me.

The ritual became sacred. Three minutes of clarity. Two focused priorities. One human connection. That was how my shifts began to *work for me*, not against me.

The next thing I needed was a way to see the whole day at a glance, not just one moment at a time.

## The Brain Sheet That Saved Me

Early on, my notes looked like a battlefield sticky note, half-scribbled times, arrows pointing in every direction. My preceptor Valsa laughed once, gently:

"If you can't read your brain sheet, how will your brain follow it?" That day, I went home and redesigned it. I drew four clean columns:

## Assessments. Meds/Times. To-Do/Calls. Family/Education.

It seemed simple, but it changed everything. The new layout became my second brain. I could glance down and see an entire shift in one view what needed to happen, what could wait, and what I needed to say to families before they left for the day.

A few weeks later, the nurse manager noticed it at the nurses' station. "This is neat," she said. "Mind if we photocopy it for the new grads?"

That quiet validation meant more than she knew. It wasn't just about paper it was proof that structure could turn panic into control. To this day, I tell my new nurses: *Your brain sheet isn't just notes; it's your safety net.*

Once my thoughts were organized on paper, I started looking for ways to make the most important details stand out.

## Color Cues

I'm not an artist, but I learned the power of color fast. Blue for assessments, red for high-risk meds, green for follow-ups. I started circling anticoagulants and insulin in bright red pen. The visual cue slowed me just long enough to double-check dosage and patient ID.

Once, that tiny pause saved me. I almost administered the wrong insulin type the names were similar, but the dose didn't look right. That red circle caught my eye. My stomach dropped. I stopped, checked, and found a transcription error. The patient never knew how close the miss came and that was exactly the point.

Color became more than decoration; it was my quiet guardian.

But even with good notes and color cues, I still needed something to slow me down in the moments that mattered most.

## Micro-Pauses

Nursing moves fast. But safety lives in the seconds you *don't* rush.

Before pushing a med or co-signing an order, I practiced what I called my "two-breath rule."

- **Inhale:** Verify the five rights- patient, medication, dose, route, time.
- **Exhale:** Reassess readiness- vitals stable? alert? allergies rechecked?

Two slow breaths. Less than five seconds. But those seconds changed everything.

One night, I was giving IV morphine to a post-op patient. He looked slightly pale, breathing shallow, but vital signs were within range. I almost proceeded. Then I paused, inhaled, exhaled, reassessed and something in my gut said *wait.* I called my preceptor. We rechecked. His O2 sat had dipped to 88%. That small pause, that single breath, prevented harm.

Since then, I've never underestimated silence. Sometimes the safest sound in nursing is the absence of hurry.

All these small habits taught me a humbling truth about confidence and control.

## System, Not Perfection

There's a myth that good nurses just "have it together." The truth? Good nurses have *systems.*

They know when to breathe, when to delegate, when to pause before charting. These habits don't make the work easier they make it survivable.

By the time my first year was halfway through, those tiny routines built a quiet fortress around my confidence. I could handle rapid changes without spiraling, because my process was stronger than my panic.

The systems didn't remove the pressure they redistributed it.

They became the scaffolding that let me stand taller, steadier, ready for whatever the next shift demanded.

But even the strongest personal systems could only take me so far; the real magic happened when they connected with the strength of the team.

## Teamwork Makes You Faster and Safer

Teamwork became the second pillar of my growing stability. Nursing, I learned, isn't sustained by individual brilliance it thrives on collaboration. You can be the most technically skilled nurse on the floor, but without the support of your team, even the smallest task can feel like climbing uphill with weights on your shoulders.

The patient care technicians were often the unsung heroes of my shift. They were the first to notice subtle changes, the first to answer a call light, and the first to lend a hand when I was juggling more than I could carry. Their quiet vigilance filled gaps no single nurse could cover alone.

One especially hectic morning, the unit was bursting with new admissions. IV pumps beeped from every corner, families lingered with anxious eyes, and the air felt thick with urgency. As I juggled three post-op patients, one of the PCTs, **Angela**, rushed toward me.

"Room 215 looks off," she said quickly. "He's breathing faster than earlier."

Her tone was firm but calm the voice of someone who *knows.* I followed her immediately. The patient's color had changed, his pulse ox dipping into the 80s. We called for help, raised the head of the bed, and started oxygen. Within seconds, the team gathered like a well-rehearsed symphony. Respiratory therapy, the charge nurse, and even the physician rounded the corner in what felt like moments.

When it was over, and the patient stabilized, Angela exhaled deeply.

"Good catch," I told her.

She smiled, brushing it off. "That's what we do."

That moment reminded me that listening to the team isn't optional it's essential. Leadership in nursing doesn't always come from a title; often, it comes from awareness and courage.

Later that week, during shift report, I mentioned Angela's quick thinking to the charge nurse. The recognition wasn't grand, just a nod and a few words of thanks but the way Angela's eyes lit up stayed with me. It reminded me that acknowledgment is a form of advocacy, too.

Each "thank you," each acknowledgment of someone's work, built a bond that made us stronger. Gratitude, I realized, is more than politeness it's glue. It holds teams together when exhaustion and tension threaten to pull them apart.

## How Trust Is Built on the Floor

It's easy to say, "teamwork matters," but real trust is forged shift by shift, in small, unseen moments.

Trust is the nurse who runs to your room when your patient's IV infiltrates mid-infusion, without waiting to be asked. Trust is the PCT who double-checks vitals on a confused patient because *something didn't feel right.* Trust is the respiratory therapist who quietly adjusts the vent settings, notices your relief, and gives you a thumbs-up on their way out.

These gestures, unrecorded in the chart, form the invisible scaffolding of safety.

When I was new, I hesitated to ask for help. Pride whispered that I should manage on my own. I worried that needing assistance made me look weak or unprepared. But the truth is, the most competent nurses I've met aren't the ones who do it all alone they're the ones who *delegate well and collaborate better.*

One evening, knee-deep in a new admission, another patient pressed the call bell for pain medication. My charting window blinked red with an overdue documentation warning. My pulse quickened. Before I could decide what to do first, **Sara**, one of the senior nurses, appeared beside me.

"I'll cover your admission labs," she said, already slipping on gloves. "You go manage your patient."

Relief flooded me so fast I almost teared up. "Thank you," I whispered.

She smiled. "We've all been there."

That night, after the handoff, I sat in my car and thought about that small act. She didn't rescue me out of pity she helped because she understood the unspoken rule of nursing: *we rise by lifting each other.*

The next day, when a new nurse looked panicked during her first rapid response, I didn't hesitate. I stood beside her, helped with her patient, and later told her the same words Sara told me: "We've all been there." The circle continued.

Teamwork, I realized, wasn't only about sharing tasks it was about sharing *grace.*

## Gratitude as Leadership

There's a quiet kind of leadership that doesn't come with a badge. It's the nurse who checks in on the night shift before heading home. The one who refills a glove box for the next person. The one who whispers, "You've got this," during a code.

In those early months, I made it a point to thank people by name. "Thanks, Mike, for catching that lab," or "Appreciate you, Angela, for noticing those vitals." Saying their names gave weight to the thanks it turned routine appreciation into recognition.

One afternoon, our unit had three discharges and two admissions back-to-back. Everyone was stretched thin. The charge nurse was fielding calls while the techs cleaned rooms. I saw **Monique**, another nurse, handling a difficult family conversation with patience that I envied. When things calmed, I pulled her aside.

"You handled that beautifully," I told her.

She looked at me, surprised. "Really? I felt like I was stumbling the whole time."

"Maybe," I said, "but your calm gave them permission to breathe."

She smiled, and for the rest of the shift, her posture changed shoulders back, eyes lighter. That's the power of acknowledgment. In a job where exhaustion often overshadows achievement, being seen can be a lifeline.

## Night Shift Lessons

On night shifts, teamwork takes on a different texture. The world outside goes silent, and inside, you become a small tribe of lights moving through dark hallways. Conversations soften. Jokes become the glue that holds you together.

One night around 2:30 a.m., my stomach growled so loudly that my patient laughed.

"You need to eat, nurse," he said, smiling.

I laughed, embarrassed. "You're not wrong."

Ten minutes later, I found a warm breakfast sandwich waiting on the counter, wrapped in foil with a note: *"Eat. You can't pour from an empty cup."*

I never found out who left it. But that gesture reminded me that teamwork doesn't just save patients it saves *us.*

## When Teams Fracture

Not every shift was harmonious. There were moments of friction sharp words in the hallway, tension during high stress, misunderstandings that lingered. Nursing can stretch people to their limits, and fatigue sometimes spills out sideways.

But I learned that how you *repair* trust matters even more than how you build it.

After one particularly chaotic morning, I realized I had snapped at a tech for something minor. The guilt followed me for hours until I finally sought her out. "Hey, I shouldn't have spoken that way," I said. "I was stressed, but that's not an excuse."

She nodded. "It's okay. We all have those mornings."

We both exhaled tension dissolved, respect intact. That moment taught me that humility strengthens teams faster than authority ever will.

## The Invisible Thread

Every nurse eventually learns that there's an invisible thread running through the unit a pulse of shared purpose that ties everyone together. You might not notice it until you need it, but when you do, it's there: steady, unbreakable, alive.

That thread is why nurses can make eye contact across a crowded hallway and communicate entire sentences without a word. It's why we instinctively step into each other's patient rooms without being asked. It's why, at the end of a grueling twelve-hour shift, we can still laugh together before heading home.

By the time I completed my second month, I realized that teamwork wasn't a soft skill it was *the* skill that determined whether a shift sank or sailed.

And the strongest teams aren't built on constant agreement they're built on *shared resilience.*

Teamwork doesn't eliminate chaos, but it transforms it. It reminds you that even when everything feels too heavy to hold, you don't have to carry it alone.

As those bonds deepened, I began to see that teamwork wasn't just physical help it was also how we spoke to one another, especially under pressure.

## Speaking the Language of the Team (SBAR in Real Life)

Working with physicians brought its own lessons. No one tells you that communication can feel more intimidating than starting an IV. The hierarchy is unspoken but palpable. You learn quickly which doctors prefer a brisk report and which want every detail. You sense who invites collaboration and who prefers compliance.

At first, I hesitated before every phone call. My notes would shake in my hand; I'd rehearse my words twice before dialing. My accent felt heavier over the line, my voice thinner. Every "Doctor, this is Pia from the step-down unit" felt like an audition for credibility.

But over time, I learned that confidence isn't about volume it's about clarity. And clarity begins with a framework.

That's when I discovered the real power of **SBAR**: *Situation, Background, Assessment, Recommendation.* It wasn't just a communication tool; it was a lifeline. It gave structure to the chaos in my head and turned anxiety into focus.

I didn't fully understand how much that framework would matter until the day it met fear head-on.

## A Lesson in Courage

One afternoon, a patient named Mr. Lu. had been admitted with congestive heart failure. He was on a strict fluid restriction and receiving diuretics. When morning labs returned, I noticed his potassium was low at 3.1. A new order for IV Lasix appeared on his chart.

My stomach tightened. Giving Lasix with hypokalemia could worsen arrhythmias. I scanned the monitor: occasional PVCs flickered on the telemetry strip. Something wasn't right.

I stared at the order, my cursor hovering. My mind whispered, *You're new maybe it's fine.* But another voice, steadier, pushed back: *You know this. Trust your training.*

I picked up the phone and called Dr. David, the attending cardiologist. He was brilliant but notoriously short-tempered one of those physicians whose presence could silence an entire hallway.

"Cardiology, Dr. David," came the sharp voice on the other end.

"Hi, Dr. David, this is Pia, the nurse caring for Mr. Lu. in 214." My heart pounded so loudly I could hear it through the receiver. "I'm calling about the new Lasix order. His potassium this morning was 3.1 and he's showing PVCs on telemetry."

There was a pause, the kind that stretches time.

"So?" he said.

I swallowed. "I'm concerned the Lasix could worsen his arrhythmia. Would you like a K+ repletion order before administration?"

Another pause. "Didn't the night team replace it?" "No, sir," I said softly. "Not yet." Silence again. Then: "Give him forty mEq oral now. Hold the Lasix for an hour. Good catch." The line clicked.

I exhaled so deeply it almost hurt. My hands trembled, but not from fear from relief. I'd done it. I had spoken up respectfully, clearly, and it had made a difference.

## Respect Earned

The next morning, Dr. David appeared on rounds. I braced myself for curt acknowledgment, but instead, he stopped at my station.

"Which one of you is Pia?" he asked.

I raised my hand.

He nodded once. "You were right yesterday. Good work."

It was three words, nothing more but they landed like validation after weeks of self-doubt. The team around me smiled. That brief exchange changed everything about how I carried myself.

From that day forward, Dr. David sought my updates first. He'd ask, "What's the plan for 214?" or "What's your take on that rhythm?" And though his tone was still brisk, there was a note of respect woven into it a recognition that I wasn't just executing orders. I was *thinking.*

That moment taught me one of the hardest lessons in nursing: **advocating for your patient sometimes means stepping into discomfort.** You won't always be liked for it, but you'll always be right to do it.

## SBAR in Motion

After that experience, I became intentional about every physician interaction. Before calling, I'd breathe once, glance at my notes, and mentally format my thoughts:

- **Situation:** Why I'm calling, urgent, concise.
- **Background:** Diagnosis, relevant history, meds.
- **Assessment:** What's changed, vitals, symptoms, labs.
- **Recommendation:** What I believe needs to happen.

The clarity it created was powerful. It wasn't just about me speaking; it helped doctors *listen better.*

A few weeks later, during a busy night, I had to call the hospitalist about a patient with worsening confusion and low blood sugar. My tone was calm, my notes clear, my voice steady.

"Doctor, this is Pia from step-down," I said. "I'm calling about Mr. R., diabetic, admitted for sepsis. His blood glucose is now 49, he's diaphoretic and slurring words. I've given oral glucose per protocol, starting D10 IV now. Do you want to modify his insulin order or hold sliding scale for tonight?"

The hospitalist's voice softened immediately. "Thank you, that's exactly the information I needed. Hold insulin, keep monitoring. You did the right thing."

I hung up smiling not because I had followed the algorithm perfectly, but because I had found my voice within it.

## The Emotional Aftermath

What SBAR really gave me wasn't a script it was *permission to sound competent before I felt it.*

The more I used it, the more natural it became. Even outside of physician calls, I used the same mental structure with coworkers and families.

Situation: *"Your dad's blood pressure dropped a bit."*

Background: *"He's on new medication today."*

Assessment: *"We're monitoring closely and adjusting his fluids."*

Recommendation: *"We'll recheck in thirty minutes. I'll update you right away."*

The same clarity that eased communication with doctors began to ease patient anxiety too. I realized that communication isn't just information it's reassurance.

## Finding My Voice

One evening, a newer nurse shadowing me confessed, "I hate calling doctors. I always sound stupid." I smiled.

"You should've heard me my first month. I rehearsed every sentence like I was calling the President." She laughed. "So, when did that change?" "When I realized it's not about sounding perfect," I said. "It's about protecting your patient. Fear can't live where purpose stands."

That line made her pause. Later that night, I heard her making her first independent call calm, clear, confident. When she hung up, she grinned. "That actually felt good." I nodded. "That's how it starts." That was the quiet ripple of mentorship in motion the way one nurse's courage passes on to another.

## When Communication Breaks Down

Not every call went smoothly. There were times a physician snapped, interrupted, or dismissed my concern. Early on, those moments crushed me. I'd replay the call in my head for hours, questioning if I'd said something wrong.

But over time, I learned to separate tone from truth. The delivery might sting, but the message still mattered. I learned to write down what was said, clarify politely, and move on without letting pride poison purpose.

Once, after a tense exchange, my charge nurse patted my shoulder. "Don't take it personally," she said. "They trust nurses who notice. They just don't always show it well."

Her words reframed everything. I realized that speaking up isn't confrontation it's collaboration under pressure.

## The Quiet Confidence

Eventually, calling physicians stopped feeling like a performance. It became a conversation between equals. Not because the hierarchy vanished, but because I understood my role within it. When I called, I wasn't just "the nurse from 3 South." I was the patient's advocate, their eyes, ears, and steady hands. I had data, judgment, and intuition tools as essential as any prescription.

And the respect that grew from those interactions didn't just elevate my confidence it elevated patient safety. Communication, I learned, is the most powerful intervention we have.

## Reflection from the Heart

That night, after the "good catch" with Dr. David, I went home, sat on my couch, and finally exhaled. For the first time since arriving in the United States, I didn't feel like I was trying to prove that I belonged. Instead, I knew I had earned it. I thought of my son, Liam, half a world away. How proud he would be to know his mother had found her voice not just in a foreign language or a foreign country, but in the language of *courage.*

And that realization changed everything about how I saw myself as a nurse. I wasn't just learning to communicate. I was learning to *stand tall in my own words.*

With my voice growing steadier, the next challenge was learning how to move through each day without losing myself in the rush.

## Pacing, Prioritizing, Protecting

Nursing isn't a race; it's an endurance event wrapped in constant sprints.

You can't control the pace of the hospital, but you can learn to control *your rhythm inside it.*

Early on, I realized that time management wasn't just about efficiency it was about safety. When I rushed, I missed things. When I slowed down intentionally, I saw more, understood more, connected more.

That's when I built my personal framework: the **4 Ps** that became my daily compass:

## Patient safety, Physician updates, Pharmacy, and Paperwork.

### 1. Patient Safety First

Every shift begins and ends with safety. It sounds simple, but it's the foundation of everything we do.

During my first few months, I used to think of safety as a checklist: allergies, ID band, bed alarms, side rails. But I learned that safety also means *awareness* reading the room, catching the subtle changes before they become emergencies.

One morning, I walked into Room 216, and my patient an elderly man recovering from surgery looked "off." His color was paler, his breathing shallow. Nothing on the monitor screamed danger yet, but instinct whispered otherwise.

"Are you feeling, okay?" I asked gently.

He nodded weakly but couldn't find words. I

reached for his hand cool, clammy. I quickly took vitals: blood pressure dropping, heart rate rising. I called for help, and within minutes, we were initiating a rapid response. He stabilized after fluids and evaluation.

Later, the physician said, “Good catch. The monitor didn’t show it yet.”

That’s when I realized: safety isn’t only in the machines it’s in your intuition, sharpened by presence.

Every nurse has that moment the one where your quiet observation changes the outcome. You don’t always get recognition for it, but it builds a deep confidence inside you that no compliment ever could.

## 2. Physician Updates

Communicating with physicians became its own rhythm, especially as my patient load grew.

The more I practiced SBAR, the more I saw the power of timing.

A well-timed update could prevent a problem from snowballing. A delayed one could turn a manageable issue into an emergency.

Once, a patient’s urine output had decreased sharply during my shift. I noted it, but the labs weren’t back yet. It would have been easy to wait. But something about the trend the IV fluids, the blood pressure, the lab delay tugged at me. I paged the physician anyway.

He came within minutes, assessed, and ordered new labs and imaging. The patient was developing acute kidney injury. Early intervention prevented transfer to the ICU.

That day taught me that updates aren’t interruptions they’re early interventions.

Every time you pick up the phone, you're not being "that nurse who calls too much." You're being the advocate who notices.

And sometimes, the physician learns from you, too. Collaboration works both ways.

## 3. Pharmacy and Meds

If nursing has a soundtrack, it's the steady beeping of IV pumps. Medications anchor much of our day and our mental load.

Early in my career, I treated the med pass like a sprint: grab, scan, go. I wanted to be efficient, to finish on time. But I learned the hard way that speed without strategy invites error.

So, I started building small systems within the bigger system.

I color-coded high-alert meds on my brain sheet red for anticoagulants, yellow for insulin, blue for opioids. I created what I called *pause points* small intentional stops before critical steps.

One night, I was about to administer IV potassium. Everything seemed correct the right patient, right order, right time. But my "pause" habit kicked in. I checked the central line order again it wasn't there. The patient only had a peripheral IV. That pause saved her from a painful infiltration.

My heart raced afterward, not from fear, but from gratitude for the lesson that safety lives in slowness.

Every time I double-checked, every time I paused for two breaths, I was building invisible armor around my patients and myself.

## 4. Paperwork (a.k.a. the Patient's Story)

If you ask most new nurses what they dread most, they'll say charting. And I get it. The documentation feels endless boxes to click, flowsheets to update, notes to sign.

But one day, during handoff, I watched how a veteran nurse used her charting like a story. Her report wasn't a checklist; it was a narrative that made sense of the patient's journey.

"She came in with pneumonia, afebrile now, but still tachy at rest," she said. "Lung sounds improving. Family very involved. She eats better when her daughter feeds her."

It struck me that her documentation didn't just record facts it reflected *care.* It was organized, intentional, and human.

From then on, I changed my mind set: charting wasn't bureaucracy it was storytelling in data form. The chart was the voice of the nurse when the nurse wasn't there.

So, I created time blocks for it: after rounds, before lunch, before handoff. Ten minutes per patient, non-negotiable. I called it my "chart and breathe" time because typing became a moment to reflect.

If you think about it, the chart is where your accountability and your compassion meet on paper. It's proof you noticed.

## Batching Tasks Without Losing Presence

Batching became my survival skill.

I learned to combine assessments, medication checks, pain reassessments, and line flushing into one efficient pass. It wasn't about cutting corners it was about conserving energy for what truly mattered.

Instead of running room to room like a pinball, I moved with purpose. When I entered a room, I was fully there not halfway in my next task. Patients can sense when you're rushing. They can feel when you're divided.

I remember one morning when I slowed down intentionally. I sat beside a patient while taking vitals, asked about her family, and made eye contact instead of glancing at the monitor. She smiled and said, "You're the first nurse who didn't look in a hurry."

I finished that room five minutes later than usual, but the rest of my shift flowed smoother. Her calm made me calmer. That's the paradox of nursing: when you slow down just enough to connect, everything else moves faster.

## Protected Five Minutes

By my third month, I added another ritual my "protected five minutes."

Right before handoff, no matter how busy the shift had been, I'd carve out five minutes to scan each chart, walk through each room, and mentally tie loose ends.

Five minutes to check IV sites.

Five minutes to ensure pain scores were updated.

Five minutes to glance at orders and labs one last time.

It became my safeguard against the regret of realizing, too late, that something was missed.

Once, during a chaotic day, I almost skipped that final check. But habit pulled me back. As I walked into one room, I noticed the patient's IV infiltrating swollen, cool to touch. I stopped the infusion and replaced the line before report. It could have caused serious pain if left overnight.

That moment reaffirmed my belief that time management in nursing isn't about finishing faster it's about *finishing fully.*

## Learning to Protect Yourself, Too

There's one more kind of protection nurses forget: protecting *yourself.* Protect your back stretch, lift correctly, ask for help. Protect your peace take breaks, hydrate, breathe. Protect your boundaries you can care deeply without carrying every story home.

I used to think self-care was indulgent, but I've learned it's discipline. The nurse who rests returns sharper. The nurse who breathes leads better. The nurse who protects her energy protects her patients.

You can't pour from an empty cup, but you can refill it quietly, shift after shift.

## Reflection

By the end of my third month, I had found my rhythm not perfect, not effortless, but mine.

The hospital still moved fast, but I moved with intention. The chaos didn't vanish; it harmonized. The alarms, the footsteps, the codes, the calls they became the soundtrack of a life lived in purpose.

I wasn't the new nurse gasping to keep up anymore. I was the nurse who paced, prioritized, and protected not only others, but herself.

That's what finding footing really means: not avoiding the storm but learning to stand steady in the rain.

And just when you start to feel steady, nursing has a way of sending a storm to test everything you've built.

## When Things Go Sideways

No matter how organized or prepared you are, there will be days when the universe decides to test every system you've built. That's the day your plan collapses under the weight of reality.

It usually begins quietly the calm before the storm. A steady morning, coffee still warm, your shift flowing just the way it should. And then, without warning, the floor tilts.

It was late in the afternoon, about two hours before shift change, when it happened. One of my patients, Mr. R., a soft-spoken man admitted for a GI bleed, pressed his call bell. His voice crackled through the intercom: "Nurse… I don't feel good."

Something in his tone made me hurry.

When I entered the room, he was pale the kind of pallor that makes your stomach tighten before your brain can name the reason. His eyes were unfocused, sweat glistening on his forehead.

"Sir, are you in pain?" I asked, pressing the call light for backup with one hand while grabbing the blood pressure cuff with the other.

He tried to answer, but his words came out slurred. The monitor flashed: **BP 82/46. HR 118.**

My adrenaline spiked. *This is it,* I thought. *Stay calm. Move with purpose.*

"Can you grab a liter of normal saline?" I called out to the PCT who had just stepped in. "And page the provider STAT GI bleed, hypotension."

The next few minutes unfolded in fragments rapid, vivid, unforgettable. I raised the head of the bed slightly, started a second IV line, and drew stat labs with shaking but steady hands. I could feel my pulse in my throat, but my training took over.

"Hang the fluids wide open," I said. "Get me a pressure bag." The charge nurse appeared at the door. "Rapid response is on the way."

Within moments, the room filled respiratory therapy, another RN, the resident. We moved like a well-rehearsed orchestra, each person knowing their cue. Someone connected the suction. Someone called for blood. Someone else printed the latest labs.

And then silence broke through the noise. The kind of silence that only comes when everyone in the room is focused on one heartbeat.

The blood pressure crept up. 90. Then 96. Then 102. Mr. R. opened his eyes, voice barely above a whisper. "Am I okay?" I smiled, even as sweat trickled down my back. "You're safe. We've got you."

When the rapid response team left, I stood by the sink, gloves still on, heart pounding in my ears. My hands shook slightly, the adrenaline refusing to let go. I caught my reflection in the metal faucet flushed cheeks, tired eyes and whispered the words I always said after moments like this:

"Thank You, Lord. For guiding my hands."

## The Aftermath

The shift continued. Another med pass, another charting session, another family question. But I wasn't the same nurse who started that morning.

That event changed how I saw chaos. Before, I feared it now, I respected it. Crisis, I realized, doesn't build your skills; it reveals them.

Later that evening, when things calmed, I replayed every second in my head: what went right, what could have gone better. I noticed how teamwork had flowed without words, how my voice had stayed steady despite my heart's rhythm racing.

The old me would have gone home replaying only the mistakes the seconds I hesitated, the words I stumbled over. The new me chose gratitude. Gratitude that training had kicked in. Gratitude that the patient was stable. Gratitude that I was learning.

That night, before I left, I checked on Mr. R. one more time. His color was better; he smiled weakly. "Thank you," he said.

I squeezed his hand. "You scared us a little, but you're doing better."

He chuckled softly. "Guess I gave you some excitement."

I laughed the kind of tired, genuine laugh that comes only after crisis gives way to calm.

## When the Adrenaline Fades

No one talks enough about what happens *after* the code, *after* the crisis. The adrenaline that once sharpened your focus begins to fade, leaving exhaustion and quiet self-doubt behind. You walk into the break room, sink into a chair, and feel the weight of what almost happened. You look down at your hands the same hands that started IVs, held pressure, and comforted and realize how thin the line can be between stability and disaster. That's when the real work begins: the *emotional debrief.*

Some nurses talk it out right away; others carry it quietly until they can process it alone. I've done both. That night, on my drive home, I replayed the sound of the monitor alarms, the flash of red on the screen, the way the team had moved. And I whispered again, "Thank You." But I also said something else I hadn't said before: "I'm proud of myself."

It felt strange, almost selfish, to say it out loud. But that moment of self-recognition mattered. Nurses are quick to blame themselves when things go wrong and slow to credit themselves when things go right. That night, I decided to balance that scale.

## Small Misses, Big Lessons

Not all lessons come wrapped in crisis. Some arrive quietly a small oversight, a missed documentation, a gentle correction from a mentor.

One evening, I forgot to reassess and document pain after giving a narcotic. My preceptor's voice was calm but firm:

"Documentation protects you and your patient."

At first, I felt embarrassed, even defensive. But later, I understood what she meant. Nursing isn't about perfection it's about accountability. Every note you write, every time you verify a med, every time you double-check an order, you're not just covering yourself you're preserving a story of care.

I began keeping a small notebook my *lesson log.* Each page started with a simple header: "Today I Learned." Sometimes it was technical ("Always label your lines before transport"). Sometimes it was emotional ("Don't skip lunch, hungry nurses make hasty choices").

Over time, those entries became my personal curriculum proof that mistakes can be teachers when met with humility instead of shame.

## The Importance of Debriefing

After every high-stress event, our charge nurse encouraged debriefing. It wasn't always formal; sometimes it was just a few of us leaning against the nurses' station, sharing what went well and what we'd do differently.

"What did we learn?" she'd ask.

That simple question turned fear into growth. It created space for honesty without judgment.

We'd laugh at the chaos, sigh at the exhaustion, and always end with gratitude. Sometimes it was as small as, "Thank you for grabbing that IV so fast." Sometimes it was as big as, "We did good today."

Those debriefs reminded me that no matter how heavy the day, no nurse carries it alone.

## Faith, Fear, and Forward Motion

That night, after the GI bleed crisis, I came home, showered, and sat on the edge of my bed with wet hair and tired eyes. My mind replayed everything the alarms, the teamwork, the relief.

I thought of my son, Liam, back home, and how every decision I made here every long shift, every learned lesson was for him.

The fear that had once paralyzed me as a new nurse had transformed into faith not blind faith that things would always go right, but grounded faith that *I could handle them when they didn't.*

Faith, I realized, doesn't erase fear; it gives it context. It says, "Yes, this is scary, but you've survived scarier."

And nursing will test that faith repeatedly every code, every heartbreak, every loss. But it also rewards it every recovery, every smile, every quiet thank-you that reminds you why you stayed.

## The Calm After

When things go sideways, it's easy to see only the chaos. But over time, you start to see something else the grace hidden inside it.

Grace in the hands that move instinctively.

Grace in the teammates who show up without being asked. Grace in the patient who lives to say, "thank you." The moments that shake you the most often shape you the most. They reveal who you are when everything is on the line. And if you look closely, those are the moments that whisper: *You're not just surviving nursing anymore. You're becoming it.*

As my skills and systems grew, another lesson emerged one that had less to do with tasks and more to do with my heart.

## Boundaries, Civility & Courage

As I grew steadier on my feet, I began learning another kind of nursing skill one no textbook could teach: how to protect my energy without hardening my heart. It's easy to think that skill and speed are the only things that matter, but the truth is, you cannot sustain compassion without boundaries. A nurse who gives endlessly without protecting her own space will eventually run dry.

## The Art of Grace Under Pressure

There were moments when kindness felt like a battle. Some colleagues dismissed me gently, others sharply a comment about my accent, a joke about "foreign training," an assumption that my education was somehow less. In the beginning, I swallowed it all. I told myself they didn't mean harm. I smiled, nodded, and kept working.

But silence can become a weight. Each unspoken word settled somewhere deep until it started to change the way I carried myself. I realized that dignity, like compassion, must be actively protected. One quiet afternoon, when someone joked that "English must be my second language," I simply said, "Yes, and I'm proud of that. It means I can care for patients in two languages."

The hallway went silent for a beat, then laughter softened into something like respect. That small exchange didn't just correct a stereotype it reclaimed my space. I learned that boundaries don't always sound like confrontation; sometimes they sound like calm truth.

## Courage in the Everyday

Courage isn't only for emergencies. It lives in small, steady acts:

- Saying "No" when someone asks you to cut corners that could endanger safety.
- Speaking up in huddles when a patient's needs are overlooked.
- Admitting when you don't know something and choosing honesty over pride.

Each of those moments builds invisible muscle. They don't make headlines, but they redefine how you see yourself. I used to think bravery meant being loud. Now I know it's about being clear.

There was a morning report where a senior nurse rolled her eyes as I presented a patient summary. My voice trembled at first, but I kept going. I focused on the data, not the judgment. When the attending nodded approvingly, I realized something powerful respect isn't requested, it's *earned in consistency.*

You don't have to prove your worth to everyone. The right people will see it in how you show up, shift after shift.

## The Weight of Emotional Labor

No one talks enough about the emotional labor of nursing. You can hold the hand of a dying patient at noon, comfort a grieving family at one, and still chart every intervention by two. You absorb more than the human heart should, and yet you keep moving.

I remember one patient, Mrs. D., who was dying of metastatic cancer. Her daughter refused to leave the bedside. Every time I entered the room, she'd ask, "Can you promise she won't die today?"

There are no right words for that question. I wanted to give her peace, but truth was the kinder gift. "I can't promise that" I said softly. "But I can promise she won't be alone."

That day, I learned that courage isn't always about doing sometimes it's about *being present* in unbearable moments. We don't fix pain; we witness it with grace.

## Learning When to Step Back

There were days I took on too much. I stayed late to help everyone, volunteered for extra shifts, said yes before thinking. It felt noble until it became numbing. I'd come home so drained I could barely eat yet still feel guilty for not doing enough.

Burnout doesn't announce itself; it creeps in disguised as dedication.

One evening, after three back-to-back shifts, I forgot to remove a patient's telemetry box before discharge. It was caught before the patient left, but the embarrassment hit hard. Valsa, ever the voice of wisdom, pulled me aside.

"Pia," she said, "you give too much without pausing. Even batteries need recharging. You can't pour from an empty cup."

Her words stayed with me. Rest is not selfish; it's stewardship. It protects the nurse, the patient, and the purpose.

## Boundary Statements that Build Respect

Through experience, I developed a few boundary phrases that kept me both professional and kind:

- "I want to give you my full attention. Can I finish this safety check and come right after?"
- "I hear your concern. Let's review the order together to be sure we're aligned."
- "I prefer to discuss feedback privately so we can focus on solutions."

Those simple sentences created space not distance. They let me stay in control of my responses without closing my heart.

Boundaries, I learned, are not walls. They are *fences with gates* strong enough to protect, flexible enough to let care in.

## The Balance Between Assertiveness and Civility

In the hospital ecosystem, emotions run high. A missed medication, a delayed lab, a frustrated family it's easy for tempers to flare. I once watched a nurse snap at a tech in front of others. The room fell quiet. Later, I approached her gently and said, "We're all under pressure, but kindness keeps the team intact."

The next day, she apologized to the tech. It reminded me that civility isn't about being nice; it's about maintaining the environment where care can thrive. A culture of respect doesn't happen by policy it happens by example.

When I became calmer, others mirrored it. The tone of my voice could de-escalate an entire shift. I began to understand leadership long before I had a title.

## Choosing the Higher Ground

There were still moments that tested me a doctor dismissing my input, a colleague gossiping, a patient's relative yelling in grief. But I learned to choose the higher ground, not because it was easier, but because it was necessary.

When someone criticizes unfairly, silence can be powerful. When someone underestimates you, excellence is the best reply. Over time, consistency becomes louder than defense.

Courage, I discovered, is not just about speaking up it's also about *how* you speak up. You can be firm without being harsh. You can advocate without antagonizing. Nursing calls for both tenderness and steel and the wisdom to know when to use each. Now it's your turn to notice where your own footing is growing stronger.

## Reflection

As I walked out of the hospital one evening, the sunset reflected on the glass facade, casting long orange shadows across the parking lot. My body ached, but my heart was light. I had survived another day not by perfection, but by presence.

That's when I realized: finding your footing isn't only about mastering skills it's about standing in your truth.

## Reflections

1. When was the last time you spoke up for yourself or your patient? How did it change you?
2. Which part of your work drains you most and what boundary could protect that space?
3. How can you balance grace and firmness when communicating under pressure?

As you keep growing, these simple practices can help you protect both your patients and your own spirit.

## Survival Tips

- **Grace is strength under control.** Use it deliberately.
- **Silence can be power** use it to listen and disarm, not retreat.
- **Protect your energy** as fiercely as you protect your patients.
- **Rest is part of professionalism.** You can't care well if you're depleted.
- **Speak truth calmly**; consistency will earn more respect than defense ever could.

## Closing Thought

Boundaries are not the opposite of compassion; they are what keep compassion sustainable. The nurse who honors her limits becomes the one other can depend on. And that more than speed or skill is what defines true courage in this calling.

## Notes

*(Use this space to write your reflections, affirmations, or personal reminders about courage, self-respect, and emotional balance. You can revisit these pages after challenging shifts to ground yourself again.)*

As I grew braver in protecting my own energy, I also began to see how much courage it takes to bridge the spaces between different cultures, languages, and ways of seeing the world.

—✦—

# CHAPTER 4

# Culture Shock and Communication

*"The limits of my language mean the limits of my world."*
*— Ludwig Wittgenstein*

Once I felt steadier with the clinical flow anticipating the day's rhythm, managing assignments, and handling admissions and discharges without drowning another challenge surfaced, one I hadn't fully prepared for. It wasn't medications, procedures, or documentation. It was people. Culture, language, and communication became the new mountains I had to climb.

The first mountain surprised me most: how much I was saying before I ever opened my mouth.

## Speaking Without Words

I quickly realized that knowing English isn't the same as communicating in a way that builds trust. My accent wasn't the barrier it was the subtleties of how I carried myself.

In the Philippines, lowering my gaze or avoiding direct eye contact signaled respect. On the unit, I noticed puzzled looks when I spoke without meeting a patient's eyes. In American culture, steady eye contact signals honesty and confidence. Without it, people feel uneasy.

The realization hit harder than any exam ever had. I had studied pharmacology and anatomy for years, yet no one had prepared me for how body language could shape care. Gestures, tone, even pauses carry meaning.

I reflected on how much of my idea of "American communication" had come not from textbooks but from TV. Growing up, I watched *MTV*, *Alfie*, *Friends*, and *Perfect Strangers*. From my living room in the Philippines, I absorbed bits of U.S. culture, the humor, the open gestures, the easy banter, the way people spoke so directly and confidently.

I imagined that was how everyone in America talked witty, fast, and effortlessly sure of themselves. But reality was different. Real conversations were layered with vulnerability, emotion, and context. What felt natural on screen sometimes felt awkward in person. One afternoon, while explaining a plan of care to a family, I caught myself looking down at the chart instead of at their faces. Their expressions told me they felt unheard. My intention was humility; what they perceived was distance.

That evening, I sat in my car replaying the interaction. I thought about how easily good intentions can be misread. If I wanted my patients to trust me, I had to meet them where they were not where I came from.

So, I practiced. Before entering each room, I took a single breath and whispered to myself, *Look at them. Meet their eyes. Be present.*

At first it felt staged. I was hyper-aware of every nod, every pause, every smile. But over time it became natural not a fixed stare, but steady, respectful contact that reassured my patients and colleagues that I was fully engaged.

One morning, a patient's wife clasped my hand and said, "You have kind eyes. I feel calm when you talk." That simple remark stunned me. All I had done was maintain gentle eye contact, but to her, it meant safety.

Gradually I noticed patterns: how Americans valued small talk, how a light joke could melt tension faster than clinical precision. Back home, silence was politeness; here, silence felt awkward. Learning to fill that silence sometimes with humor, sometimes with empathy became a bridge across cultures.

That small shift taught me something profound: communication isn't only about words; it's about presence. What is respectful in one culture can be misinterpreted in another. Adapting doesn't mean abandoning who you are it means building bridges so you can truly connect.

As weeks passed, I noticed subtle changes. Patients opened more readily. Families were calmer during explanations. Colleagues who once seemed distant started including me in quick jokes and hallway conversations. My words hadn't changed much, but my energy had. I was no longer translating language; I was translating connection.

But the deepest test of communication came when my clinical training and a patient's deepest beliefs stood on opposite sides of the same decision.

## The Power of Understanding

The hardest lesson came with a patient who had sickle-cell anemia. Their blood counts dropped dangerously low, and the team recommended a transfusion. To me, it was a straightforward, lifesaving intervention. The patient, a devout Jehovah's Witness, refused.

"I'm worried," I said gently. "Your labs are very low. A transfusion would help your body recover." "My faith doesn't allow it," they replied, unwavering. Their family echoed the same resolve.

For days, I cared for them managing pain crises, monitoring labs, watching numbers fall. Between tasks, we talked not always about medicine, but about life, family, and faith. A closeness formed beyond nurse and patient.

Each night I prayed for a miracle, wrestling with a truth I didn't want to accept. My training told me to save; their belief told me to respect. When the patient died, it shattered me. I performed post-mortem care with trembling hands, whispering a quiet prayer as tears slid down my face.

Deep down, I knew this wasn't failure it was respect. Communication isn't always about persuading; sometimes, it's about honoring choices, even when they break your heart.

In school, we were taught to advocate for life, prevent harm, save when possible. No textbook prepared me to advocate for autonomy for a patient's right to make a choice that went against everything my training urged me to do.

Driving home that night, headlights blurred by tears, I realized communication is a mirror of empathy. Sometimes it means speaking; other times, it means surrendering to silence and presence. Healing takes many forms. Honoring a patient's belief can be a form of healing, too.

That loss changed me forever. It shaped the educator I later became the one who reminds new nurses that advocacy is not about control; it's about compassion wide enough to hold difference.

After that, I could no longer see conversations as routine; each one felt like a bridge I was either building or breaking.

## Bridges Built on Listening

From then on, I approached each patient with fresh eyes. I asked more about what mattered to them. I listened not just to their words but to their values and fears. The daily hurdles remained: misunderstood jokes, unfamiliar slang, hand gestures with unexpected meanings. I once told a patient to "move forward a bit," meaning scoot up in bed; he laughed and asked if I was "proposing a life plan." We both laughed until the tension dissolved. Humor, I discovered, was a universal language.

Other times, missteps humbled me. A colleague once said, "Can you grab the blue top from the Pyxis?" I spent ten minutes searching for an actual blue-topped container, not realizing it was shorthand for a lab tube. She found me eventually and said kindly, "We've all been there." Instead of embarrassment, I felt belonging.

Little by little, I built bridges. I repeated back what I heard to confirm. I practiced new habits until they felt natural. I learned when to explain gently, when to advocate firmly, and when to sit in silence honoring another human being.

I discovered that communication is as critical as clinical skill. Without it, no amount of knowledge can build trust. With it, even the hardest conversations can become moments of healing even when outcomes aren't what we hope for.

Communication is an art that demands vulnerability, patience, and humility. It requires more than a well-rehearsed explanation; it requires a genuine connection. I began listening not just to what patients said, but to what they didn't the pauses, the hesitations, the quiet moments when fear sat between us.

Listening became my superpower. It turned strangers into collaborators. And in the noise of alarms and orders, listening became the softest but strongest form of leadership.

In time, I realized that listening was only the beginning; what I did with what I heard was its own kind of language.

## The Language of Empathy

Some days, communication looked like translating jargon into comfort. Other days, it meant standing silently by a patient as they cried, knowing my presence mattered more than words. Sometimes, it was sharing a small laugh bridging distance with humor that reminded us of our shared humanity.

Language and culture are powerful. They can divide or unite, create misunderstanding or open the door to healing. As an immigrant nurse, being bilingual wasn't just about speaking two languages; it was about living between worlds interpreting not only words, but emotions, values, and perspectives. I learned to read between lines, to sense hesitation behind a patient's "I'm fine," to catch gratitude in a family's quiet nod.

Every encounter became an opportunity to practice cultural humility. I learned to ask before assuming, to listen before judging, to respect before reacting. One evening, a Spanish-speaking patient smiled when I greeted her with a simple "Buenas noches." Her eyes lit up. "You tried," she said. It wasn't perfect Spanish, but it was perfect humanity. The beauty of nursing isn't in knowing everything; it's in staying open enough to keep learning.

By several months in, the culture shock that once made me anxious transformed into curiosity. Instead of fearing misunderstanding, I saw it as an invitation to grow. Each conversation awkward or effortless became a chance to deepen both skill and empathy. At the bedside, I learned that communication is more than exchanging information; it's about helping people feel seen, heard, and valued.

That realization changed not only how I cared for patients, but how I carried myself in every part of life.

Now I invite you to look at your own conversations and the stories they're telling.

## Reflections

1. When have you felt misunderstood because of how you expressed yourself? What did it teach you?

2. Recall a time you cared for someone whose beliefs differed from your own. How did you balance respect and duty?
3. Which habits or cultural norms from your upbringing shape how you communicate?
4. How can you use silence as a tool for connection rather than discomfort?
5. What does "presence" look like in your daily practice?

*Take a few minutes to write. Reflection is the foundation of cultural humility.* As you grow in that humility, a few simple habits can help you navigate culture shock and communication with more grace.

## Survival Tips

- **Listen before you speak.** Silence often reveals what words cannot.
- **Ask instead of assuming.** Curiosity prevents misunderstanding.
- **Respect differences.** Beliefs aren't barriers; they're doorways to understanding.
- **Let empathy be your language.** When words fail, compassion translates.
- **Stay teachable.** Every patient and colleague expands your understanding.
- **Clarify early repeat back** what you heard; confirmation builds trust.
- **Remember: communication** includes tone, posture, and presence.
- **Humor heals.** A light heart can bridge even the widest gap.

Taken together, these practices turn everyday conversations into opportunities for connection instead of conflict.

## Closing Thoughts

Culture shock and communication will test you in ways textbooks never describe. You will stumble over differences, miss jokes, and sometimes face the heartbreak of choices you cannot change. Yet these moments reveal the **heart of nursing.**

Communication isn't perfect language it's listening deeply, respecting differences, and building trust across barriers. When you can do that, you are not just a nurse with skills; you are a nurse who connects. And connection is where healing begins.

## Notes

*(Use this space to reflect on moments when you built or struggled to build connection across cultures. Let it be your reminder that every misunderstanding can become a lesson in empathy.)*

________________________________________

________________________________________

________________________________________

________________________________________

________________________________________

________________________________________

But even as communication became easier at work, I soon learned that the hardest conversations were the ones I had with myself when the shift was over.

# CHAPTER 5

# Balancing Work and Life

*"You can't pour from an empty cup, but you also can't refill one you never put down."*

Once I began to settle into the unit's rhythm, another challenge surfaced one no orientation manual had prepared me for. It wasn't IV pumps, medication schedules, or documentation. It was what happened **after** I took off my scrubs and left the hospital.

I learned quickly that nursing doesn't end when the shift ends. The day followed me home like an echo that refused to fade. Alarms still rang in my mind long after I clocked out, stitched into my heartbeat. Patients' faces lingered behind my eyelids. The grief of losses trailed me into the quiet of my apartment.

Fatigue lived not just in my muscles but in my soul. Some nights I dropped my bag by the door, too tired to cook or speak. The silence felt heavy a strange contrast to the beeping, paging, and rushing I'd left behind. My body left the hospital, but my mind stayed there, looping through tasks and what-ifs. Nursing, I realized, doesn't have an "off" switch. And the more the job followed me home, the more I realized I was carrying far more than just clinical responsibility.

## The Weight of Carrying Two Worlds

Even as exhaustion thickened, life outside the hospital still called for me bills to pay, groceries to buy, loved ones waiting on the other side of the world. I had left home to build a better life, but in doing so I was living two lives at once.

Every text from family carried joy and ache. A message from my son, Liam, a voice note filled with laughter was both calm and reminder. His childhood was happening in real time while I watched through a screen. I whispered promises to photos on my fridge: *Someday soon, we'll be together.*

The loneliness wasn't constant; it came in waves. It surfaced in quiet moments after saving a patient's life or after losing one when there was no familiar hand to hold. I learned that homesickness isn't just missing a place; it's missing the version of yourself that existed there.

Each morning, I put on my scrubs like armor. Each night I peeled them off like a second skin. I was a nurse by profession, but survival had become an art form.

But beneath that daily balancing act was a deeper struggle one I couldn't ignore once I began losing patients.

## The Hidden Cost of Caring

Some of the hardest moments came from the patients I couldn't save. Protocols were followed, orders double-checked, teamwork flawless and still, sometimes, it wasn't enough.

There was the elderly patient whose body slowly surrendered, despite every intervention. There was the young man whose collapse sent shockwaves through the unit. There were the quiet vigils by the bedside, holding a hand as life slipped away.

Those moments didn't stay in the hospital. They followed me home, into dreams and dinner tables, into long walks where my mind replayed each sequence, searching for a different ending. I learned that grief doesn't need permission to visit.

Compassion, I discovered, has a cost. Every life you touch leaves a fingerprint on your heart. The trick is not to erase those fingerprints but to carry them gently, without letting them bruise you.

At first, I thought strength meant forgetting. Later, I learned strength meant remembering and still returning the next day to do it all again.

And in the quiet moments between shifts, the heaviest ache wasn't the job it was distance.

## Motherhood Across Miles

Every nurse carries a private story behind the badge. Mine was motherhood divided by oceans.

Each night, after back-to-back twelve-hour shifts, I came home to an apartment that echoed with absence.

The clock struck midnight as I video-called Liam. He would be eating breakfast, sunlight streaming through the kitchen window back home. "Mom, I drew you!" he'd say, showing a stick-figure nurse with a big smile.

I smiled too, though tears blurred my screen. Distance has a sound it's the pause between hello and goodbye when the call ends, but your heart keeps listening.

That longing fueled me. It reminded me that every shift, every sacrifice, was a bridge I was building toward him. Loving from far away required sacrifices I counted not just in emotions, but in numbers.

## The Math of Survival

Survival required more than grit; it required math. Rent, bills, groceries every dollar was a decision. I budgeted on sticky notes, counting coins before sleep. "Musts, Goals, Life," I labeled three columns. Under Musts: rent, utilities, rice, and transit. Under Goals: savings for Liam, visa renewals, and emergency funds. Under Life: a single small joy flowers from the corner market, a book, or jasmine tea.

The spreadsheet of sacrifice was my quiet triumph. Each month I survived proved that hope could live on a paycheck stretched thin.

My apartment was small, but it held the scent of home garlic frying, a rosary by the bed, a photo of Liam by the window. Every detail reminded me: I was building something worth the ache.

Still, even the strongest purpose can crumble without rest, and my body began to demand what my pride had ignored.

## Rest as Resistance

I once believed rest was a luxury. Nursing taught me it was a necessity.

On days off, guilt whispered that I should study, clean, catch up on errands. But my body begged for stillness. Resting became rebellion a declaration that my worth wasn't tied to constant motion.

Sleep became sacred. I learned the rhythm of blackout curtains, white-noise fans, and silenced phones. I treated naps like prescriptions and honored rest like a duty to my patients.

Because a tired nurse is a risk, and caring for myself was another form of caring for them.

But even rest wasn't enough, I needed people who understood this world without explanation.

## The Power of Connection

Connection kept me afloat. Calls with Liam anchored me; his laugh reset my heart. Conversations with fellow nurses reminded me that my struggles weren't mine alone.

We found humor in chaos laughing at tangled IV lines and misplaced brain sheets. Potlucks after long stretches of shifts felt holy. We shared meals, stories, and survival. Those nights reminded me that community was medicine, too.

We cried together after codes, celebrated small wins like clean audits or early discharges, and reminded one another that burnout didn't define us belonging did. And even with community around me, I needed small, personal rituals to steady myself.

## Micro-Rituals of Healing

Healing wasn't grand or dramatic; it lived in the small rituals:

- Tea before bed, steam curling like a prayer.
- A walk around the block, just to remind my lungs that the world was larger than the hospital walls.
- Writing three lines of gratitude one for myself, one for my patients, one for tomorrow.

Gratitude didn't erase exhaustion, but it reframed it. It turned survival into meaning. Still, meaning is not enough when your nervous system stays stuck in hospital mode long after the shift ends.

## When the Shift Follows You Home: A Decompression Plan

I couldn't silence the alarms in my memory, but I could teach my body that danger had passed.

## The 5-5-5 Reset (15 minutes at the door)

- **5 breaths:** Inhale 4, exhale 6, signal safety.
- **5 minutes:** Gentle movement: roll shoulders, stretch neck, loosen tension.
- **5 minutes:** Transition ritual: shower, change lighting, make tea, step outside. Mark the end of the shift.

### Then two grounding questions:

1. What did I do right today?
2. What will I do differently next time?

These small rituals stopped my mind from replaying the entire day. They reminded me that the shift was over and I had done enough. Even with decompression, I learned there was a difference between being tired and being emptied out completely.

## Compassion Fatigue vs. Burnout (And Why It Matters)

- **Compassion Fatigue:** Your empathy is tired. You feel numb toward suffering you once felt deeply.
- *Antidote:* connection and meaning share one patient story that moved you today.
- **Burnout:** Your system is overloaded. Work feels hopeless or detached.
- *Antidote:* boundaries and balance reduce extras temporarily, protect days off like medication windows.

Recognizing the difference saved my career more than once. Fatigue needed rest. Burnout needed re-alignment. And realignment often starts with words we're afraid to say, the boundaries that protect us from collapsing under the weight of caring.

## Boundaries You Can Say Out Loud

Early on, I thought boundaries were selfish. Then I realized they were a **safety measure.**

- “I can help after I finish this medication pass.”
- “I need ten minutes to chart safely; I’ll update you right after.”
- “I’ve reached my safe limit for extra shifts.”

With time, these boundaries didn’t distance me from my work they allowed me to show up more fully.

## Closing Thoughts

Balancing work and life as a nurse are not about perfection it’s about presence.

Some days, you’ll feel like you gave everything at work and have nothing left at home. Other days, you’ll leave work early enough to cook, call family, or simply breathe. Both days count.

Balance isn’t static; it shifts with every patient, every season, and every choice to pause. Remember: your life is more than your job, but your work is also part of your life’s purpose. Hold both gently.

As you learn to hold both your work and your life with care, these simple practices can help you stay balanced and whole.

## Survival Tips

- **Create rituals of transition.** Don’t bring the hospital home. Simple actions like changing clothes, lighting a candle, or journaling can signal your mind that the shift is over.
- **Prioritize sleep and nourishment.** They’re not luxuries they’re survival tools.

- **Schedule "nothing" time.** Protect at least one block a week where you do not plan or produce anything.
- **Keep one joy within reach.** Whether it's tea, music, or a favorite show, joy is not optional; it's restorative.
- **Ask for help before you break.** Strength isn't silence. Find your people early mentors, peers, family and lean on them.
- **Remember who you are outside the badge.** You existed before nursing, nurture that person, too.

## ✏ Notes

*(Use this space to reflect on how you currently balance work and life. What boundaries do you need to set? What brings you peace outside nursing?)*

______________________________________________

______________________________________________

______________________________________________

______________________________________________

______________________________________________

______________________________________________

And as I learned to balance my life outside the hospital, I began to confront another truth, every nurse must face growth often begins where mistakes are made.

# CHAPTER 6

# Mistakes and Lessons Learned

*"Failure is not the opposite of success; it's part of success."*
*- Arianna Huffington*

No one becomes a nurse without making mistakes. We may not always talk about them, but they happen to all of us. In school, perfection feels like the standard. In practice, we learn we're human. The real test isn't whether you make a mistake it's what you do next.

In my first months on the step-down unit, mistakes felt like shadows: following every shift, every med pass, every chart I signed. I carried a constant fear of failure of harming a patient, of being reported, of confirming what some already suspected: that as a foreign-trained nurse, I wasn't "good enough." I wanted Liam to look at me with pride, not doubt. My first lesson came on a morning when everything moved too fast for comfort.

## The Medication Mix-Up That Could Have Been

One morning with a full assignment and call bells ringing, everything happened at once. Doctors were rounding, new orders were printing, families wanted updates. In the rush, I nearly gave a blood pressure medication to the wrong patient.

Two men with similar last names were waiting for their morning meds. I had already scanned the first pill when I noticed the date of birth didn't match.

My heart stopped.

"Wait," I said softly, pulling the cup back. I rechecked the wristband, label, and chart. Relief washed over me: the mismatch was caught in time. The entire moment lasted less than a minute. To me, it felt like an eternity.

That night, I replayed the scene repeatedly. I pictured Liam and reminded myself that every patient is someone's child, someone's family. From that day forward, I promised to slow down, no matter how hectic it became. Seconds spent confirming identity are seconds well spent.

Mistakes caught early are not proof of incompetence they're proof of vigilance. But not every mistake announces itself so loudly some appear quietly, tucked inside the chart.

## When Documentation Tells the Truth

Not all mistakes announce themselves with alarms. Some whisper.

One afternoon, I documented a narcotic administration but failed to return and chart the reassessment.

Discharges, admissions, and competing priorities pushed it out of my mind. On review, it looked as if I hadn't followed up at all.

My preceptor pulled me aside. Calm, firm: "If it isn't charted, it isn't done."

The words landed harder than a reprimand. I realized that compassionate, skilled care can vanish without a record. Documentation isn't busywork; it's truth, protection, and continuity. That night I stayed late to double-check my notes. Over time, I made it a ritual: **my care will not vanish unrecorded.**

Charting became my way of saying, *"I was here. I cared. I acted."*

Still, some of my hardest lessons had nothing to do with medications or notes they came from moments when I stayed silent.

## The Power of Clarifying

Other times, the mistake was silence. During a call, a physician rattled off orders quickly. I caught most of them but not all. Pride kept me from asking to repeat. I told myself I'd figure it out later. I missed a key instruction. Thankfully, another nurse clarified before harm occurred, but shame burned. I practiced new words after that:

"Doctor, let me read that back."

Awkward at first, lifesaving in practice. Humility is safer than pride; silence isn't respect, it is risk. I started carrying a small notepad for calls. Simple change, huge difference.

Now, whenever a nurse hesitates on the phone, I remind them, "Ask again. You're not questioning their authority you're protecting their patient." Silence taught me consequences but so did fear. And nothing tested that fear like my first rapid response.

## The Rapid Response That Changed Everything

My first Rapid Response etched itself into memory. A patient's blood pressure dropped, breathing grew shallow. The room transformed into urgency. The team flooded in voices overlapping, monitors beeping. I froze. Hands shaking, I gripped the IV pole to steady myself. My mind screamed *do something,* but fear pinned my body.

After the patient stabilized and transferred to ICU, shame sat heavy. A senior nurse found me later. "Everyone freezes during their first rapid," she said kindly. "Next time, you'll know what to do. What matters is you learned." She was right.

The next time a rapid was called, muscle memory surfaced. I managed the pump, tracked vitals, handed supplies. Still nervous but no longer frozen. Fear had turned into focus. That shift from hesitation to action was the first time I truly felt myself growing into the role. That lesson came full circle when I found myself on the other side catching someone else's near miss.

## Paying It Forward

Soon after, I experienced the other side. I walked into a room and saw a colleague preparing an IV medication that I remembered was ordered IM. "Wait," I said gently. "Let's double-check the MAR."

She looked surprised, then relieved. Together, we corrected it before harm. For the first time, the weight of my earlier lessons lifted into something more powerful: **vigilance.**

My mistakes had sharpened me not only for my own practice, but to protect my patients and support my team. I thought of Liam. I hoped that if he were ever a patient, a nurse would pause, double-check, and step in. But the hardest part wasn't the mistake itself it was facing the emotional weight that came afterward.

## Owning Mistakes Without Letting Them Own You

Each mistake or near-miss stung in the moment and followed me home to the hum of the refrigerator and the weight of fatigue. I held a cup of tea, stared out the window, and thought of my son's laughter. Every lesson made me stronger, safer, more capable.

I learned:

- Mistakes don't define me; my response does.
- Owning errors builds credibility faster than hiding them.
- The nurses I admire aren't perfect; they're honest, accountable, and compassionate with themselves.
- Mistakes aren't proof that I don't belong. They're part of how every nurse grows.

I began each shift with a new mindset not *I must be perfect*, but *I must be present.*

I breathed before reacting, slowed down in chaos, and turned errors into reflection. Fear of failure softened into respect for responsibility. Fear kept me cautious; reflection made me wise. Wisdom doesn't come from doing everything right it comes from surviving what you didn't and choosing to keep going.

Over time, I realized that mistakes don't live in isolation they live in the culture surrounding them.

## The Culture of Safety: Speaking Up Without Shame

The units that thrive aren't the ones without errors they're the ones where nurses can talk about them safely. Creating a "speak up" culture means:

- **Normalize reflection, not blame.** Every debrief should end with "what did we learn?" not "who messed up?"
- **Mentor transparency.** Leaders should model humility by sharing their own early-career errors.
- **Encourage second checks.** Peer verification is collaboration, not criticism.
- **Build psychological safety.** New nurses should never fear retaliation for honest mistakes reported promptly.

When safety becomes shared, fear turns into accountability, and accountability builds trust. To turn these lessons into growth, I began practicing intentional reflection.

## Reflection Journal Exercise

Try this after a hard shift:

1. **Describe what happened.** (Stick to facts, not judgment.)
2. **Identify the emotion.** (Fear? Guilt? Embarrassment?)
3. **List what you controlled and what you didn't.**
4. **Name the lesson.** (What safeguard will you add next time?)
5. **Write one affirmation.** ("I am learning. I am growing. I am still worthy.")

Mistakes become wisdom when written down. Reflection transforms regret into resilience.

Now I invite you to explore your own experiences with honesty and compassion.

## Reflections

1. Recall a mistake from your early practice. What did it reveal about your habits, and how did you change them?
2. How do you respond when a colleague is struggling? What helps you step in with courage and kindness?
3. What can you do this month to strengthen a culture of safety where nurses can speak up without fear?
4. What sentence of self-compassion do you need to hear after a tough day?

Write honestly. Reflection turns guilt into growth. And as you continue to grow, these simple habits will help you stay grounded, safe, and resilient.

## Survival Tips

- **Slow down to stay safe.** Seconds saved by rushing can cost safety.
- **Ask, clarify, confirm.** Repetition isn't weakness, it's wisdom.
- **Own your mistakes.** Accountability builds trust.
- **Document thoroughly.** The chart is the story of your care.
- **Let fear teach you, not limit you.** Channel it into focus and checks.
- **Debrief early.** Don't let the weight of "what if" grow overnight.
- **Celebrate small recoveries.** Catching an error before it reaches a patient is a success, not a shame.

With time, these truths shape not only how you practice, but how you see yourself as a nurse.

## Closing Thoughts

You will make mistakes. Every nurse does. You'll feel fear, shame, and doubt. Don't let those moments crush you let them teach you. Let them sharpen your attention, deepen your humility, and build your resilience.

One day you'll look back and see those missteps for what they were: stepping-stones that made you safer, stronger, and wiser.

Nursing will humble you, but it will also mold you into someone braver than you imagined.

## Notes

*(Use this space to document lessons learned, near-miss reflections, and affirmations for growth.)*

And as I learned to face my mistakes with honesty, I noticed something just as powerful the people around me were shaping me just as much as the lessons themselves.

# CHAPTER 7

# MENTORS, FRIENDS, AND FOES

*"We become ourselves through the people who steady us, stretch us, and sometimes stand against us."*

The step-down unit was relentless. From the first hour of my shift to the last, I felt as if I was running just to keep from falling behind. Alarms blared, call bells echoed, and voices carried through the hallways in a constant stream of orders and requests. My scrubs clung stiffly to me, my badge looked too new beside those of seasoned nurses, and my hands trembled each time I logged into the computer. I felt like an outsider, unsure whether I would ever find my place in a world that moved faster than I could breathe.

Just when I wondered whether I would ever find my footing, someone stepped into my story with calm, steady guidance.

On one of my first shifts, **Valsa** was the charge nurse. She was a senior nurse of Indian background calm, composed, with a presence that steadied everyone around her. Thin gold bangles chimed softly as she moved, her steps measured and unhurried. Her accent carried warmth that softened her instructions, and her words calmed even my most frantic thoughts. That morning, she looked at me kindly and said, "Stay close today. We will make it work." Her reassurance felt like a lifeline.

Throughout the day she guided me with a balance of firmness and gentleness. When an IV pump wouldn't stop alarming, she came to my side, patient as she explained the sequence of buttons to silence it.

"Do not rush," she said, tapping the keypad with sure fingers. "These machines like to test us."

When I double charted a vital sign and panic rose in my chest, she showed me how to correct the entry calm and matter of fact. Errors weren't the end, she reminded me; they were opportunities to learn.

Valsa taught lessons beyond the clinical. One evening, a patient's family became frustrated their voices sharp as they questioned the care their loved one was receiving. I froze, afraid of making things worse. Valsa stepped beside me, steady and kind.

"Listen first," she whispered. Then she acknowledged their fears, addressed their concerns, and set gentle boundaries without escalating the conflict. Watching her, I realized nursing is not only tasks and procedures, but also presence, compassion, and the ability to stay calm when emotions run high. Families often need reassurance more than answers. They want to know they are seen.

But not every lesson came wrapped in kindness. Some came through sharp words that cut deeper than expected.

Not all colleagues were supportive. Some left me questioning myself. One of the hardest moments came from **Nurse Lily**, a senior nurse. I had been floated to the ICU to cover until staff could be arranged. I felt a spark of pride that my charge nurse trusted me. When Lily heard, she narrowed her eyes and said flatly, "You are too young for this. You do not belong in there."

Her words stung. She was Asian too, and I had expected some measure of solidarity. Instead, her tone carried judgment. It felt as if my youth, my accent, and my Filipino background automatically disqualified me. I held my tongue and swallowed the anger and shame. Deep down I made a quiet promise: **I would prove her wrong.**

For days, her words echoed each time I stepped onto the unit: *you do not belong in there.* I began to second-guess everything each medication I prepared, each assessment I charted, each answer to a physician. Lily had no authority over me, yet her disapproval carried weight because she represented what I wanted to become: seasoned, confident, unshakable. It took time and mentors like Valsa to quiet that voice.

Competence, I learned, isn't proven by convincing others; it is built through consistency, compassion, and determination. I took Lily's skepticism and turned it into focus. I studied harder, paid closer attention, and sought feedback from people I trusted. Every nurse has someone who believes in them and someone who does not. Both can teach you, but only one deserves your energy.

Thankfully, for every voice that made me doubt myself, there was another that helped carry me forward.

**Sharon**, a patient care technician, became one of my anchors. Her energy seemed endless moving from room to room with fresh linens, vital signs, and water trays. Despite her workload, she always found a smile or a word of encouragement.

One morning, overwhelmed by a full assignment, a new admission, and multiple call bells, I froze in the hallway mind blank, hands full, heart racing. "I will take this one, nurse," Sharon said with a quick wink, slipping into a ringing room. "Go catch your breath."

Her kindness saved me that day. Without Sharon and others like her, I would not have survived those first months. Nursing is not a solo job it is a team effort among nurses, technicians, secretaries, and physicians. At the end of grueling shifts, when we finally collapsed into chairs, Sharon would say, "We made it." Those simple words reminded me I was not alone.

Friendship in nursing often grows in the spaces between chaos: a shared glance during a code, quiet laughter in a supply room, a small gesture after a hard loss. One night, after a patient passed unexpectedly, the silence was heavy. Sharon found me at the nurse's station eyes red, voice unsteady. She did not offer advice. She handed me a cup of water and sat beside me until I could breathe again. That is friendship: presence, not platitudes.

And beyond nurses and technicians, I learned that physicians, too, played a quiet part in shaping who I was becoming.

Among physicians I saw a spectrum. At first, many barely acknowledged me the new nurse with the accent and the uncertain voice. Over time, some noticed. **Dr. David**, a cardiologist known for brisk rounds, did not strike me as encouraging. For weeks I felt invisible at the edge of his group. Then one morning, after I monitored a patient with irregular rhythms, he turned and asked, "Nurse, what do you think?"

My heart pounded, but I reported my overnight observations. He gave a short nod. "Let us continue the current plan." A small exchange, but to me it meant everything. Respect arrives slowly, built through vigilance and consistency, and one day it appears without fanfare.

The contrasts were stark Valsa's steady mentorship, Sharon's friendship, Dr. David's earned recognition, and Lily's doubt that became my challenge. Each shaped my journey. Some lifted me, some tested me; all made me grow. Nursing is learned through people as much as through policies. Every interaction becomes part of your foundation. **Mentors show what to emulate. Friends show what to cherish. Foes show what to overcome.**

In quiet moments after long shifts, when exhaustion pressed heavy, I thought of **Liam**. His small voice on the phone "How was your day, Mama?" reminded me why I endured. I wanted him to know his mother was strong, that she did not give up in the face of judgment or fear. Every patient, colleague, harsh word, and kind gesture became part of the story I would one day tell him. Mentors reveal who you are; friends remind you to extend compassion to yourself; critics teach endurance. **Self-belief is not handed to you; it is built shift by shift, challenge by challenge.**

## Mentor Moments I Keep

- "Stay close today. We will make it work." *Safety is learned shoulder-to-shoulder.*
- "Do not rush; the machine is not the patient." *Slow is smooth; smooth is safe.*
- "Listen first." *People calm when they feel seen.*

## What I Learned from a Friend

- A cup of water and quiet company can be more healing than speeches.
- Laughter in the clean utility room is a pressure valve.
- "We made it" is a blessing, not a cliché.

## What a Foe Taught Me

- Doubt from others can become discipline in you.
- Not every voice deserves equal space in your mind.
- You don't need permission to belong. You prove it by caring well.

These moments good and painful became the compass points of my early career.

## Reflections

1. Which mentors shaped your growth, and what qualities made their guidance meaningful?
2. Recall a criticism that pushed you to grow. How did you turn it into motivation?

3. Who brings balance to your day's encouragers, truth tellers, quiet supporters?
4. What single sentence of self-belief do you need to keep near your badge?

Write freely. Reflection turns experience into gratitude.

As you take these lessons into your own practice, let these reminders steady you.

## Survival Tips

- **Find mentors early.** Seek those who lift you with honesty and patience.
- **Let criticism refine you, not define you.** Meet it with grace.
- **Cherish your team.** No nurse thrives alone.
- **Earn respect quietly.** Consistency and integrity speak loudly.
- **Remember your why.** Purpose outshines doubt.
- **Practice presence.** Before answering tension, breathe and *listen first.*

In the end, every relationship during your first year leaves an imprint some gentle, some harsh, all transformative.

## Closing Thoughts

People you meet in your first year will shape you in ways you cannot predict. Let mentors teach you, let friends sustain you, and let critics sharpen your resolve. In the end, every voice kind or cruel becomes part of the chorus that transforms you into the nurse you are meant to be.

## Notes

*(Use this space to map the people who shape you mentor, friend, challenger and the lessons they bring.)*

But even with mentors guiding me and critics sharpening me, there was still one journey I had to make on my own the slow, quiet journey toward believing in myself.

# CHAPTER 8

# Growing Into Confidence

*"Confidence is not something you find; it's something you build every time you refuse to give up."*

Confidence does not appear overnight. It builds slowly, in pieces, through small victories that add up to something solid. At first, I doubted myself with every step. My hands trembled with a syringe, my voice wavered when I called a physician, and my heart raced whenever an alarm sounded. Every beep echoed my fear a reminder that one mistake could unravel everything I had worked for.

I wondered if I would ever feel comfortable in my uniform. I envied senior nurses who seemed to glide through chaos with calm precision. How did they move with such certainty while I felt like I was fighting to keep my head above water?

Over time something shifted. Confidence did not arrive with fanfare it crept in quietly, moment by moment. It appeared in the seconds between panic and poise, in the way my hands began to move when I needed them to, and in the calm, I found while facing what used to terrify me. That lesson became real on a morning when fear and skill collided in a single breath.

## The Moment Fear Met Competence

One busy morning, a patient with congestive heart failure struggled to breathe. His oxygen saturation dropped, his face turned pale, and the room filled with the fragile tension between control and crisis. For a split second the old fear returned, and my instinct was to look for someone more experienced. Then something inside me whispered, *you can do this.*

I raised the head of the bed, checked the tubing, listened to his lungs, and called the physician. My report was steady and clear. I gave the vitals, explained my findings, and offered a recommendation. When the physician agreed, I hung up and realized my voice had not shaken.

I had acted like a nurse.

That quiet milestone was everything. Confidence had begun to bloom, not in the absence of fear, but because I moved through it.

But confidence isn't built from crises alone, it grows even more in the quiet, everyday wins that no one else sees.

## The Small Victories That Built Me

Confidence also grew in the smallest triumphs.

I remember the first IV I started on the first attempt the flash in the chamber, the patient saying, "That did not even hurt." Warm pride washed over me. It wasn't only skill; it was proof.

I remember catching a critical potassium trending down and calling immediately. The physician thanked me for vigilance, and I realized attention to detail saves lives.

I remember discharging a patient on my own, reviewing medications and instructions, and hearing, "Thank you, nurse." For the first time, the title felt like it belonged to me.

These weren't grand moments. They were ordinary tasks done with care but together they built a bridge from self-doubt to self-trust. Confidence, I learned, is built quietly behind the scenes, one correct action at a time.

And slowly, those small victories began to change not just how I worked, but how I carried myself around others.

## When I Became the Voice of Reassurance

A few months after orientation, a new nurse joined the unit. She reminded me of myself wide-eyed, overwhelmed, terrified of making a mistake.

She whispered, "I don't think I can do this."

Without hesitation I said, "You will get through this. You know more than you think. Take it one patient at a time."

Only later did I realize I was no longer seeking reassurance; I was giving it. That was the moment I knew something within me had changed. Confidence doesn't always shout. Sometimes it whispers, reminding you that you've grown in ways you haven't measured.

But confidence didn't erase mistakes, it simply changed how I faced them.

## Learning to Stand Tall After Mistakes

Confidence also changed my relationship with mistakes. It didn't mean I stopped making them; it meant they no longer destroyed me.

Early on, a missed documentation note or a confusing order would haunt me for days. With time I learned to see those moments as lessons about vigilance, humility, and grace. Confidence wasn't the absence of fear it was the ability to act despite it.

Fear still came, as it always does, and each time I met it, it loosened its grip.

Confidence is not built in ease; it's shaped in recovery. Every time I made an error, reflected, and corrected it, I was proving to myself that I could fall and still rise safely.

And with each recovery, I found courage to use my voice in ways I never had before.

## Finding My Professional Voice

I began to recognize the power of my voice. At first, I was afraid to question physicians, worried I would seem incompetent or disrespectful, so I spoke too softly. As confidence grew, I spoke up with respect and assurance.

Sometimes my suggestions were dismissed; other times they were acknowledged. I practiced saying, "Doctor, let me repeat that back to you," to ensure clarity. It felt awkward at first, then it felt professional.

During rounds, Dr. David asked for my observations. I reported fluid balance, rhythm, and response to diuretics. He listened, nodded, and said to the team, "Let us continue the current plan."

For months I had felt unseen as though my accent and uncertainty marked me as small. In that moment I felt respected, valued, and recognized as a contributor to care.

Respect is not handed to you. It is earned, layer by layer, through consistency, accuracy, and quiet excellence.

Yet confidence wasn't only about speaking up it was also about staying strong when the emotional weight of nursing pressed hardest.

## Endurance as a Form of Confidence

Confidence was not only about skill or interactions; it was about enduring the emotional toll. There were nights I came home too exhausted to eat, and days when a patient's suffering followed me their faces, final words, and a family's grief echoing in my memory.

Confidence meant believing I could carry these burdens and still return the next day. It meant trusting that I had the strength to endure even when I missed my son, **Liam**, so deeply that the ache felt physical.

Sometimes, after a long shift, I called home just to hear his voice. "Mom, kamusta ka na? I miss you."

"I am okay," I would say, wanting him to hear strength to know that distance cannot break love, and that sacrifice, however painful, is never wasted.

My confidence as a nurse grew alongside my determination as a mother. Every shift, every small success, became a thread in the future I was weaving for us.

And somewhere in the middle of exhaustion and growth, the work that once felt overwhelming began to feel familiar.

## When Routine Became Rhythm

Over time patterns emerged. I anticipated needs before patients asked, recognized subtle signs of distress, and saw the look of fear before a procedure. I no longer chased the rhythm of the unit; I moved with it.

The once-chaotic beeps and alarms became a familiar symphony not pleasant, but purposeful. Confidence wasn't knowing everything; it was trusting myself to keep learning. The chaos remained, but I was not drowning.

I was swimming with intention, with belonging, with grace.

There were still hard days. Confidence did not erase short staffing, heavy loads, or complicated families but I met them with quiet conviction.

Instead of telling myself *I cannot*, I reminded myself, *I have done this before, and I can do it again.*

Each time I walked into a room, I took a breath and thought: *You are enough.*

I might not know every answer, but I knew enough to ask the right questions, to act quickly, and to comfort gently. That is the heart of nursing not perfection, but presence.

The lessons that shaped my confidence were simple, but they stayed with me.

## Lessons That Stayed

- Confidence grows slowly, built from small victories that seem ordinary at first and life-changing later.
- True confidence is not perfection; it is resilience standing up after mistakes and moving forward stronger.
- Your voice matters. Speaking up with respect doesn't create doubt; it builds trust.
- Confidence isn't the absence of fear; it's the decision to act despite it.
- Every nurse begins uncertain. The brave ones stay long enough to see certainty bloom.

Take a moment to look at your own journey, and notice where confidence has quietly taken root.

## Reflections

1. What small victories built your confidence?
2. When was the last time you surprised yourself with how much you knew?
3. Who helped you believe in yourself before you did?
4. What does confidence look like not in others, but in *you*?

Write what comes. Reflection makes growth visible. As your confidence continues to grow, keep these small but powerful habits close.

## Survival Tips

- **Breathe before you act.** Calm precedes clarity.
- **Record your wins.** Keep a "confidence log" with small victories.
- **Speak your truth with respect.** Clarity prevents conflict.
- **Don't chase perfection.** Chase progress.
- **Remind yourself daily:** You belong here.

And when doubt returns, as it always will, remember how far you've already come.

## Closing Thought

You will not wake up one morning suddenly full of confidence. It will come in small, quiet ways in an IV you place on the first try, in a moment when a physician asks for your input, in the reassurance you offer a new nurse who reminds you of yourself.

One day you will look back and realize the trembling hands and wavering voice are gone. You are no longer surviving shift to shift you are thriving.

When that day comes, pause and whisper, *you did it. You belong here.*

Caring beyond the bedside is where the science of nursing meets the art of humanity and in those quiet, unmeasured moments, you will discover the meaning of this calling.

## Notes

*(Use this space to record milestones of confidence your first success, your first "I can do this," your first thank-you that felt real.)*

And as my confidence grew, I began to understand something deeper that the heart of nursing often lives far beyond the tasks, the skills, and the bedside itself.

# CHAPTER 9

# Caring Beyond the Bedside

*"Healing is not always about curing. Sometimes it is about accompanying someone through what cannot be fixed and letting love be enough."*

## The Encounter and Emotional Discovery

When people imagine nursing, they picture IV lines, vital signs, and medications. They see nurses rushing through bright hallways, juggling orders, charting on computers, and responding to alarms. Those things are real nursing is science and skill, discipline and precision.

But the truth runs deeper. Nursing lives in the spaces between the tasks in the unseen, undocumented moments when you sit at a bedside and simply *be* with someone. It's in the quiet gestures no one teaches you: the straightened blanket, the gentle tone when delivering hard news, the stillness of your presence beside fear.

One evening, I met a woman who changed what I believed care could be. She was in her early sixties, her body fragile from pancreatic cancer. The room smelled faintly of antiseptic and lavender lotion, a small attempt to soften the clinical air. She had no family and no visitors. Her husband had passed three years earlier, and the silence in her life had grown loud.

When I entered, she looked up and whispered, "I do not know if I can do this."

No textbook had prepared me to answer that.

I sat down and took her hand. "You do not have to do this alone," I said quietly.

We sat together for nearly an hour. She told me about her husband, their house full of photographs, the daisies that bloomed each spring in her garden. She cried softly for the loneliness that followed his death. When she asked what I believed about life after death, I told her the truth: "I believe love never really leaves us. It changes form, but it stays."

I left her room changed. There would be no charting box for that hour, no line item that read *listened to fears, offered presence*. That night I understood something I had only glimpsed before nursing was never meant to be confined to procedures. It was about *humanity*.

After that encounter, I began seeing the deeper layers of nursing everywhere, quiet needs hidden behind stable vitals, unspoken fears beneath routine assessments.

## Advocacy, After-Shifts, and Reflection

After that night, I began noticing how often the truest work of nursing happened quietly, in the background.

A man recovering from cardiac surgery was stable on paper normal vitals, clean incision, good labs yet his silence was heavy. He stared out the window at the parking lot and answered, "I am fine," on repeat. *Fine* can hide pain.

I pulled a chair beside him. "Tell me what is really on your mind."

Slowly he whispered, "I am tired. I do not know if I can keep doing this." He didn't need another lab order he needed a witness. That day, I learned that listening is one of the purest forms of care.

Advocacy followed soon after. A middle-aged woman was cleared for discharge, yet something in my gut said otherwise. Her speech was slower, her movements unsteady.

"Doctor," I said gently, "I am concerned. She is dizzy and confused." He waved me off. "She will be fine." I kept my tone calm but firm. "This is not her baseline. She needs one more day."

He sighed and agreed. The next morning her blood pressure plummeted.

Advocacy, I realized, is not confrontation it's *compassion with courage*, the refusal to stay silent when safety is at stake.

After shifts like these, faces lingered as I washed dishes or folded laundry. Sometimes the grief of others mingled with my own. On those nights, I missed my son most. "Mom, kamusta ka na? I miss you." His voice wrapped me in warmth. It reminded me why I kept going not just to make a living, but to make a difference worthy of the distance. The love I carried for my son became the same love I poured into my patients: quiet, constant, unconditional.

But with that love came a weight I hadn't expected, a tenderness that felt like both a gift and a burden.

## The Privilege and Burden of Caring

Caring beyond the bedside taught me that nursing is both privilege and burden a sacred service that asks you to show up with your *whole heart*, even when it's breaking.

Not every patient will remember your name, but they will remember how you made them feel the nurse who met their eyes, who didn't rush, who sat down when everyone else stood.

Some nights I cried after hanging up my scrubs not from regret, but from the truth that healing does not always mean recovery. Sometimes it simply means peace. And peace often begins with *presence.*

When you stay beside someone through fear or grief, you offer a gift words cannot capture: the assurance that they are not alone. That is the heartbeat of nursing the sacred space between doing and being.

As you walk this path, let these truths guide and protect your heart.

## Survival Tips for Caring Beyond the Bedside

1. **Be still.** Not every problem needs a solution. Sometimes patients need silence and company.
2. **Listen with your heart.** Notice what isn't said the sighs, pauses, and tremors.

3. **Advocate boldly and respectfully.** If something feels off, speak up. Your intuition is an instrument of care.
4. **Protect your spirit.** Carry empathy without letting it consume you. Breathe, write, pray, seek sunlight.
5. **Remember your humanity.** You cannot pour from an empty cup. Rest is preparation to serve again.
6. **Celebrate unseen victories.** The moments that never get charted often matter most.
7. **Lean on your why.** When exhaustion sets in, return to the reason you began.

Now take a moment to look inward and honor the ways this kind of caring has shaped you.

## Reflections

1. Recall a moment when you offered presence instead of intervention. What did it teach you?
2. Who or what reminds you of your *why* when compassion fatigue sets in?
3. How can you protect your emotional energy without closing your heart?
4. Which small, unrecorded acts of kindness restored your faith in this calling?

Write freely. Your reflections are part of your healing. And as you continue caring beyond the bedside, hold close the moments that remind you why this work matters.

## Closing Thought

Tasks will fill your days, but moments beyond the bedside will fill your heart. IVs, medications, and vitals matter, but they are not what patients remember.

What endures is your compassion, your presence, and the gentle way you make people feel seen. Caring beyond the bedside is where the *science* of nursing meets the *art* of humanity.

Every quiet act of kindness, every hand you hold, every tear you witness, every minute you stay becomes the truest definition of healing.

These are the moments that stay with you long after the shift ends the ones that shape not only the nurse you are, but the human you become.

And as these moments shaped me, I found myself wishing someone had gently told me what I now know truths that would have eased my fears and steadied my steps.

## Notes

*(Use this space to reflect on the patients or moments that reminded you what "caring beyond the bedside" truly means. Write about how you nurture empathy, advocacy, and self-compassion in your daily practice.)*

The advice I share here was not learned in classrooms or lecture halls. It was shaped by long nights, difficult lessons, quiet victories, and the people who carried me along the way.

—✦—

# CHAPTER 10

# ADVICE TO NEW GRADUATE NURSES

*"The first year doesn't make you, it reveals you."*

## The First Year and My Dual Lens

Every nurse remembers their first year.

The badge clipped proudly to your scrubs sits beside a quiet fear: *Can I really do this?*

I remember trembling as I hung my first IV bag, double-checking every label, my heart pounding as I documented, afraid that a single wrong click could undo everything. Those memories are still vivid etched into my hands, my heart, my humility.

Time and experience softened those memories into perspective. Now, as a Nurse Residency Coordinator, I see those same fears mirrored in the residents I mentor. When I watch them clutch clipboards and whisper, *"I hope I did that right,"* I see my younger self nervous, hopeful, and unsure.

That is both the beauty and ache of this profession: it asks you to relive your beginnings each time you help someone else start theirs.

My advice does not come from textbooks. It comes from life from nights when I doubted myself, from patients whose trust demanded courage, and from residents who sat across from me with tears in their eyes, convinced they were not enough. I tell them what I wish I had heard back then: *You are not walking this path alone.*

Before you learn the skills, you must learn yourself your fears, your strengths, and the courage it takes to keep showing up.

## Learning Through Struggle

Skills will come with practice. What matters first is the willingness to try, fail, learn, and try again. New nurses often measure success by what they complete IVs on the first try, on-time discharges, perfect documentation.

These are good goals, but they can become traps. Nursing is not a checklist. It is a craft refined through repetition, reflection, and humility. Growth arrives quietly: in the steady hand that no longer trembles, in the thank-you that lands deep in your chest, in the moment you stop rehearsing every step out loud.

The confident nurse who moves with ease once stood where you stand now fumbling, uncertain, afraid of being exposed as an imposter. Experience smooths the edges, and it's born from mistakes.

I share mine freely:

- The blood pressure pill I almost handed to the wrong patient because their last names were similar.
- The charting omission that made it appear care had not been provided.
- The misheard telephone order I was too timid to clarify.

None defined me. They taught me the rhythm of accountability:

## Pause. Breathe. Verify. Own it.

A mistake corrected honestly becomes a lesson. A mistake hidden becomes a risk. Honesty is the cornerstone of trust with patients and with teams. Many residents confess errors expecting punishment but receive guidance instead. I tell them: *"You are not the first, and you will not be the last. What matters is that you spoke up before harm was done."*

That courage is the beginning of growth.

## The Power of Asking for Help

The more you speak with intention and listen with depth, the more your voice becomes one of your greatest tools. One of the hardest lessons to learn is that asking for help is not weakness it is *wisdom.* I've seen residents hesitate, hands hovering over a pump, fear whispering: *What if they think I don't know what I'm doing?* No one expects you to know everything. Pretending can be dangerous. A question asked in time prevents a crisis later. Patients are never harmed because a nurse asked for clarification. But harm has come when someone stayed silent.

Humility and confidence are partners.

It takes courage to say, *"I need a second set of eyes,"* and strength to ask, *"Can you double-check this with me?"*

When you seek guidance, you are not revealing ignorance; you are demonstrating professionalism.

You are building a bridge to your team's shared wisdom.

You will not grow alone. The nurses beside you, the mentors who steady you, and even the critics who challenge you will become part of your story.

## Teamwork: The Heartbeat of the Unit

Nursing is a collective effort. Every successful shift is a symphony of hands, minds, and hearts.

The PCT who notices a new shortness of breath. The secretary who flags a critical lab.

The respiratory therapist who catches a decline before it's too late. Each one is essential. You are never truly alone in the room, even when it feels that way.

Respect is the currency of teamwork. A simple "thank you" to the tech who empties a drain or to the clerk who tracks down a missing result goes further than you realize. Gratitude builds trust, and trust turns a unit from a workplace into a *family.*

I remind new nurses: *No one can thrive on an island.* You survive your first year not by standing out but by standing *with* others.

If I could place one final truth in your hands, it would be this confidence grows not from knowing everything, but from caring deeply enough to keep learning.

## The Emotional Toll and What It Teaches

And when the shift is over, your healing matters too. Your career will last decades, and your wellbeing must last with it. No one can fully prepare you for the emotional weight of your first year. Residents come to me after long nights, eyes swollen from tears, confidence shaken. Patients lash out. Physicians dismiss input. Families demand answers you don't yet have.

Exhaustion burrows deep. You are not failing you are *forming.*

Growth rarely feels graceful. It looks like doubt.

It looks like tears behind a break room door.

It looks like breathing through a mistake and returning the next day anyway.

Confidence is forged in friction in the long shifts that push you past your limits. The pain you feel becomes the empathy you offer. The heaviness you carry becomes the light you give.

I remember my own nights of collapse at the kitchen table; sure, I was weak. Looking back, those nights made me stronger.

They taught me the discipline of *returning* of showing up again, even when my heart felt empty.

That is the quiet miracle of nursing:

You can feel drained, and still, by morning, you rise and give again.

## Reflections

1. Which moments have shaped you most triumphs or mistakes and what did they teach you?
2. Who steadies you when the noise of the unit becomes too loud?
3. How are you caring for yourself beyond the hospital walls through rest, food, movement, or connection?

Write your answers somewhere you can revisit.

They will remind you that you are growing, even when progress feels invisible.

## Survival Tips for New Graduate Nurses

1. **Breathe before every patient room.** One steady breath reset focus. Presence matters more than perfection.
2. **Ask early and often.** Clarifying orders and processes is diligence, not incompetence.
3. **Learn your team's rhythm.** Respect every role; collaboration becomes second nature.
4. **Own mistakes, then release them.** Accountability builds trust; rumination drains energy.
5. **Protect your energy.** Hydrate, eat, and rest you cannot pour from an empty cup.
6. **Document with purpose.** Your chart is the written story of your care.
7. **Keep a gratitude note.** One win, each shift compounds into confidence.

8. **Return to your why.** Family, faith, or purpose will anchor you when you feel lost.

One day you will look back and realize you have become the nurse you once hoped you would be. Not suddenly, not perfectly, but faithfully shift by shift, lesson by lesson.

## Closing Thought

The first year will stretch you in ways you never expected. You will doubt yourself. You will question your strength. You may even wonder if you chose the right path. And yet, in those same moments, you will discover resilience, empathy, and a voice that is uniquely yours. Mistakes will become lessons. Chaos will become rhythm. Fear will turn into focus. One day, you will catch your reflection in a patient's window and see what others already see a nurse who belongs.

When that day comes, thank the version of yourself who kept showing up, asked for help, cried in silence, and refused to quit.

The real story of every great nurse is not perfection. It's *persistence.*

Use this space to gather the advice you want to carry with you, truths you want to remember on the days when the work feels heavy and the learning feels endless.

## Notes

*(Use this space to reflect on your journey as a new graduate nurse. What moments have revealed your strength? What lessons do you want to carry forward as you grow in this profession?)*

______________________________________________

______________________________________________

______________________________________________

______________________________________________

______________________________________________

______________________________________________

—✦—

# CHAPTER 11

# THE WEIGHT OF RESPONSIBILITY

*"Responsibility in nursing is not about carrying the weight alone. It's about learning how to carry it with grace."*

## The Invisible Burden

Nursing is not just a profession it is a vow, a promise written not in ink but in trust.

The moment you accept an assignment, you carry the weight of another person's life in your hands.

Outsiders cannot see it, yet every nurse knows how heavy it feels. It presses in the hum of monitors, in alarms that pierce through fatigue, and in the trembling voice of a family member asking, *"Will they be okay?"*

In my first year, I learned that responsibility in nursing is both humbling and crushing. It can feel like a mountain on your shoulders, and it is also what gives our work its sacred purpose. Responsibility is not only a duty; it is a form of love in action.

## Signing My Name

The first time I signed my name as the *primary nurse*, my pen shook. The signature looked the same, but it carried a new weight: *I am accountable for this person's life.* That single line was more than documentation it was a declaration. I was here. I acted. I took responsibility.

Years later, that quiet weight still returns every time I sign my name. Each stroke is a covenant proof that I stood in the space between life and loss and did my best to serve faithfully.

One evening, a frail man recovering from surgery asked softly, "Am I going to be okay?" I froze. I wanted to promise yes, but honesty caught in my throat. I didn't know. So, I sat beside him, took his hand, and said, "I will do everything in my power to keep you safe." That moment taught me that responsibility is not about having every answer.

It's about being present when assurance is needed most. Patients might forget your words, but they never forget your *presence.*

## When the Weight Feels Too Heavy

There were shifts when the weight nearly broke me. I carried it home like a shadow that refused to fade. One night, a young patient declined rapidly.

The team rushed in compressions, fluids, medications voices blending into a desperate symphony. Still, we lost him. I remember driving home at dawn, the sky dim, my hands shaking on the wheel. My scrubs were damp, my throat dry, my heart hollow. One question looped in my mind: *Did I do enough?* It haunted me for days.

Part of nursing is learning to carry grief without letting it devour you. You do not clock out from responsibility it follows you into your sleep, your silence, your breath. Grief, I discovered, is the shadow side of love. You cannot have one without the other.

## Learning to Prioritize

Early on, I tried to do everything perfectly answer every call light, soothe every concern, complete every task flawlessly. The pressure nearly consumed me. Gentle mentors taught me an essential art: *prioritization.* Responsibility is not doing everything at once it's doing the *right thing first.* One question became my compass: **"What will keep my patient safest right now?"** That clarity transformed chaos into structure and panic into purpose. I learned that excellence is not in doing more it's in doing what matters most.

## Advocacy as Duty

Responsibility includes speaking up when silence feels safer. Early in my career, a patient was being prepared for discharge, yet she was unstable.

Doubt whispered, *who am I to question a senior physician?* I spoke up anyway. The discharge was delayed, and the next day complications confirmed the concern. That day I understood that advocacy is not defiance it is *compassion with courage.*

To care is to speak, even when your voice shakes. True responsibility is not about authority. It is about accountability to the patient, to your conscience, and to the truth.

## Carrying Grief, Carrying Love

Responsibility means carrying *grief* and *love* in equal measure. You stand at the bedside of the dying, and you celebrate with those who heal. You witness final breaths, first smiles, and every heartbeat in between. When I lost my son, Liam, I thought of the families I had comforted. Their tears had soaked my sleeves; their pain had carved space in my heart. Responsibility does not only prepare you to hold others' grief it teaches you how to survive your own.

Alongside grief comes love: patients who thank you through tears, families who hug you in hallways, colleagues who whisper, *"You did everything you could."* that love steadies you when the weight feels unbearable. It reminds you why you chose this life.

## Reflections and Exercises

1. Recall a moment when you felt the full weight of responsibility. What emotions surfaced, and how did it shape you?
2. Write about a patient whose presence or gratitude stayed with you long after your shift ended.
3. Reflect on a time you advocated when it felt uncomfortable. What gave you courage?
4. Consider how you carry work home. What ritual, conversation, or self-care practice helps you release the weight more gently?

Take time to write without judgment. Reflection transforms burden into meaning.

## Lessons That Stayed

- Responsibility is accountability. Every signature, every chart, every act matters.
- Responsibility is presence. Silence can heal when it comes from empathy.
- Responsibility can feel crushing. Let grief carve you, not consume you.
- Responsibility requires prioritization. Do what protects life first.
- Responsibility is advocacy. Speak up it is duty, not defiance.
- Responsibility holds both grief and love. You need both to remain human.
- Responsibility extends beyond the shift. Protect your own heart too.

## Closing Thought

The weight of responsibility never vanishes.

It shifts as you grow stronger beneath it. Nursing will always demand accountability, presence, and courage. With time, the same weight that once crushed you will shape you. It will sculpt compassion, strengthen integrity, and remind you that you are not meant to carry the burden alone but to carry it *with grace.* You may still wonder, *Did I do enough?* But if you showed up, stayed present, and spoke for those who could not, then you did what nurses are called to do. And that, always, is enough.

## Notes

*(Use this space to reflect on the moments when responsibility felt heaviest — and how you carried it. What helped you move forward with grace, even when the outcome was beyond your control?)*

______________________________________________

______________________________________________

______________________________________________

______________________________________________

______________________________________________

______________________________________________

As I learned to carry responsibility with steadier hands, I also learned to carry myself. Each hard moment softened something inside me; each victory strengthened something I didn't know I had. Without realizing it, responsibility became the doorway to a deeper journey one that started long before my first shift and transformed me long after.

And when the shift is over, your healing matters too. Your career will last decades your wellbeing must last with it."

—✦—

# CHAPTER 12

# Looking Back, Moving Forward

*"Courage isn't the absence of fear; it's the quiet decision to keep moving forward despite it."*

## The Young Woman Who Left Home

When I look back at the young woman who stepped onto a plane with twenty dollars and a trembling heart, I barely recognize her.

She clutched her documents tightly, blinking back tears as she waved goodbye to her family, to the familiar streets of the Philippines, and to her son, Liam her reason for everything.

She was terrified and alone, but she carried something stronger than fear: a promise to carve a life filled with opportunities she never had.

I remember the ache of separation as I walked through immigration, the way my body trembled with exhaustion and grief the moment I landed in New Jersey. The skyline was vast and bright not hope yet, just survival.

Those early years were harsh. I signed contracts that felt confining, worked shifts that drained me, and faced doubts that echoed in every unfamiliar hallway. Some nights I cried in a tiny apartment, wondering if I had made a mistake or if I was strong enough to keep going.

But a small, persistent flame refused to go out.

Each morning, I pictured Liam's smile.

And I whispered to myself, *"For him, I will try again today."* And every day, somehow, I did.

## Becoming the Nurse I Needed

Over time, nursing became more than a job, it became a journey of becoming.

My defining moments didn't arrive with dramatic music or applause. They arrived disguised as ordinary tasks:

- The first time I advocated for a patient and was heard.
- The first full assignment I managed without panic.
- The first time a physician asked for my input and listened.
- The first time a patient said, "You made me feel safe."

These small victories built the nurse I would one day become.

Becoming a Nurse Residency Coordinator didn't happen overnight. It was the culmination of thousands of tiny steps, shifts that left me in tears, mistakes turned into lessons, and long nights where I gathered the strength to return again in the morning.

Now, when a nurse resident sits across from me with trembling hands and tear-filled eyes, convinced they are failing, I see my younger self the same fear, the same exhaustion, the same fragile hope.

I tell them what I learned the hardest way:

"These feelings do not mean you're failing. They mean you're growing."

Growth is rarely gentle. It stretches you. It breaks you open. It rebuilds you into something stronger.

Skepticism from colleagues, the loneliness of being far from home, and the pressure to prove myself all of it became the soil where resilience grew. Patients taught me compassion. Mentors taught me direction. Critics taught me endurance.

And grief the deepest, most private part of my story taught me strength.

Now, when I see a new nurse gripping a chart with trembling fingers, I smile quietly.

I know what it feels like to stand exactly where they stand to be scared, and to move forward anyway.

## Reflections

Looking back, I learned that struggle is not a sign of weakness it is the evidence of transformation. The girl who once doubted herself became a woman who leads, teaches, and advocates.

If I could speak to that younger version of myself crying alone after a thirteen-hour shift,I would tell her:

You will make it.

You will stumble and rise again.

You will cry, and those tears will water your strength.

One day, you will help others find their way too.

Every scar, every sleepless night, every moment of fear each became part of the story that shaped the nurse, the mother, and the woman I am today.

## The Lessons That Stayed

- **Your past is not a limitation**; it is a foundation. Where you came from will deepen the way you care.
- **Struggle builds character.** Hard days become strength later.
- **Courage is quiet.** It's not dramatic, it's persistence.
- **Growth takes time**. Great nurses are shaped slowly.
- **Humility and confidence can coexist.** Stay teachable and know your worth.
- **Connection heals.** No nurse succeeds alone lean on your people.
- **Love your work and love your life, too.** The care you give others begins with how you care for yourself.

## Closing Thought

If you are holding this book as a new graduate or foreign-trained nurse at the beginning of your journey, hear the words I wish someone had said to me:

You belong here.

The fear you feel is normal.

The doubt you carry is proof that you care.

Inside you are a strength that grows shift by shift, patient by patient, lesson by lesson.

One day, you will look back not only at how far you have come, but at how deeply you have grown.

And when you meet another nurse standing where you once stood trembling and brave you will tell them:

"You can do this." And in that moment, you will realize: You already have.

## Survival Tips for Moving Forward

- Honor your journey every struggle holds a lesson.
- Let reflection shape your growth, not self-criticism.
- Carry confidence gently; it grows with practice.
- Keep learning curiosity is one of your greatest strengths.
- Seek mentors and be one when the time comes.
- Protect the parts of you that make you compassionate.
- Celebrate quiet milestones they matter.

## Notes

*(Use this space to reflect on your personal journey where you started, who helped you grow, and who you've become along the way.)*

# EPILOGUE

You Were Meant for This

*"You are not behind. You are becoming."*

## The Journey Ahead

If you are holding this book, perhaps you are where I once was standing at the edge of a new beginning, afraid yet hopeful, unsure yet determined.

Maybe you are a foreign-trained nurse leaving behind family, culture, and home to build a life from the ground up. Maybe you are a new graduate stepping into your first hospital job, your scrubs crisp, your badge brand new, your hands trembling with a mixture of fear and possibility.

Whoever you are, wherever you stand, know this: you are not alone.

The road ahead will not always be smooth. There will be nights when the weight of responsibility feels unbearable, when your confidence cracks under pressure, when your heart aches for home or for a version of yourself that felt less tired and more certain.

You will cry in supply rooms. You will doubt your worth. You will question your place in this profession. And yet you will also grow in ways you cannot yet imagine.

You will save lives not only through medicine, but through gentleness. You will earn trust not only through knowledge, but through presence.

You will gain confidence not all at once, but quietly moment by moment, patient by patient, shift by shift.

Then, one ordinary day, in the midst of the hum of monitors and footsteps, you will realize something extraordinary:

You are no longer just surviving.

You are becoming.

You have grown into the nurse you once prayed you could be.

## A Promise Kept

When I began this journey, I was a separated mother with two suitcases, twenty dollars, and a heart torn between fear and hope. I left my son, Liam, with a promise that one day, these sacrifices would make sense.

I arrived in a country that did not yet feel like home, worked under contracts that tested my resolve, and faced doubts that whispered I was not enough. Still, I kept going. I showed up when I wanted to give up. I learned even when I felt behind. I cared even when my heart was breaking.

Somewhere along the way, I became more than a nurse.

I became a mentor.

A teacher.

A voice.

I carried my story, and somehow, it carried me back to myself. If I could speak to the girl at the airport clutching her passport through tears, I would say: You will build the life you dreamed of.

You will find your voice.

You will become the woman your son will one day be proud of. And if I could, I would whisper the same to you.

## A Letter to You

May this book be your companion in doubt.

May it remind you that nursing is not only about skill it is about soul.

It is the courage to care when no one is watching. The humility to admit when you do not know. The strength to rise again after every fall.

When you stand at the bedside of a patient who reminds you of someone you love, may you feel the sacredness of that moment.

When you advocate for a voice that cannot speak, may you remember that once, yours went unheard too. When you mentor another nurse someday, may you extend the same grace that once lifted you.

And when the world feels heavy, return to this truth: You are exactly where you are meant to be not perfect, not finished, but becoming.

## Looking Forward

One day, you will look back not with regret, but with quiet pride and see how far you have come. You will remember the moments that once felt impossible and smile at how they shaped your strength.

You will realize that you did not simply survive nursing's first year.

You grew through it.

You rose from it.

You became the nurse, the advocate, and the human you were always meant to be.

So, take a breath.

Straighten your badge.

Step forward.

The world needs what only you can give.

And I am here, quietly cheering for you because I know exactly how far you will go.

## Reflection Prompts

*Use these prompts for honesty, growth, and self-discovery. Journal privately, share them with mentors, or revisit them at each milestone year.*

### 1. Your Beginning

- What emotions surfaced on your first day as a nurse?
- What hopes, fears, or expectations did you carry into your first shift?
- If you could speak to that earlier version of yourself now, what would you say?

### 2. Lessons in Growth

- Recall one mistake or near miss that changed how you practice. What did it teach you?
- Which patient, mentor, or colleague shaped your compassion or confidence the most?
- What surprised you about yourself during your first year?

## 3. Balance and Belonging

- How do you care for yourself after a difficult shift?
- Which boundaries or rituals keep you grounded outside work?
- Who reminds you that you are more than your badge?

## 4. Purpose and Passion

- What aspect of nursing fills your heart with meaning?
- When did you first feel that you truly belonged in this profession?
- How will you use your voice to uplift the next generation of nurses?

Remember: Reflection is not about reliving mistakes it is about recognizing how far you have come. Every honest page becomes another layer of growth.

— ✦ —

# ACKNOWLEDGEMENTS

No journey is traveled alone. This book was born from the love, strength, and faith of the people who walked beside me through every challenge, triumph, and quiet moment of doubt.

**To John Erman Morales Obidos**- my mentor and leader. Thank you for your steady guidance, for believing in my potential when I doubted myself, and for modeling leadership rooted in kindness and wisdom. Your influence continues to shape the educator, mentor, and nurse I strive to be.

**To my colleagues, educators, and nurse residents**- you are my inspiration. You remind me every day that nursing is a calling built on courage, compassion, and lifelong learning.

**To my husband, Gerry** - your patience, love, and unwavering support have carried me through every storm. You are my home.

**To my daughter, Perrine**-your laughter is my light. Your curiosity and joy make every sacrifice worthwhile.

**To my mother, Ming**-your love has been the foundation beneath every step of my journey in the United States.

Your care for Perrine allowed me to chase opportunities I could not have reached alone.

**To my siblings Phoebe, Peter, Pam** -thank you for filling my life with joy, belonging, and warmth. Having you and your families here in the United States has made this journey whole.

**To Liam, my beloved son in heaven** this book is yours as much as it is mine. Your spirit lives in every word. You are the reason I endured, the reason I kept my promise, and the light that continues to guide me. You are my forever why.

And finally, **to every nurse new graduate, mentor, foreign-trained dreamer** this book is for you. You are proof that courage transcends fear, that compassion crosses borders, and that strength is born from service. May this book remind you that your journey matters. May it give you faith when you feel unseen, courage when you feel uncertain, and the assurance that you are exactly where you are meant to be.

# ABOUT THE AUTHOR

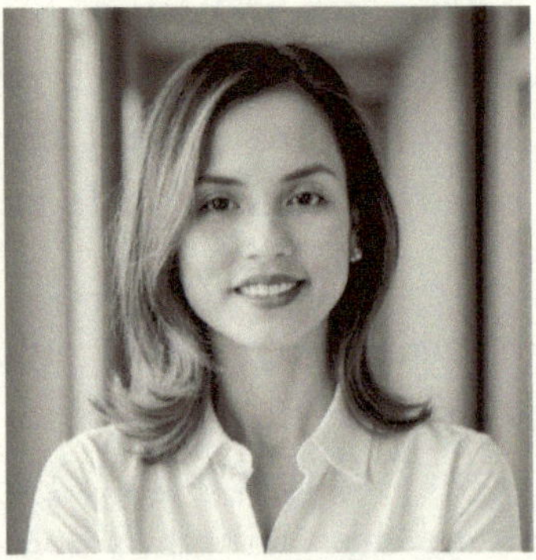

**Pia Dy, MSN, RN, PCCN** is a nurse educator, mentor, and storyteller passionate about supporting new graduate and internationally trained nurses as they transition into clinical practice.

Born and raised in the Philippines, Pia began her nursing career overseas before immigrating to the United States, where she rebuilt her life through resilience, determination, and faith.

Today, she serves as a Nurse Educator and Nurse Residency Program Coordinator, guiding new nurses from uncertainty to competence, from survival to confidence. Through teaching, writing, and advocacy, Pia continues to honor a promise she made years ago to help nurses not only make it through their first year but thrive.

Beyond her professional role, Pia is a wife, mother, and lifelong learner dedicated to wellness, leadership, and storytelling. Her work celebrates the voices of nurses everywhere their struggles, their triumphs, and their profound humanity.

www.ingramcontent.com/pod-product-compliance
Lightning Source LLC
La Vergne TN
LVHW100317210926
848480LV00003B/1153
*9798993923208*